ABC HEALTHY

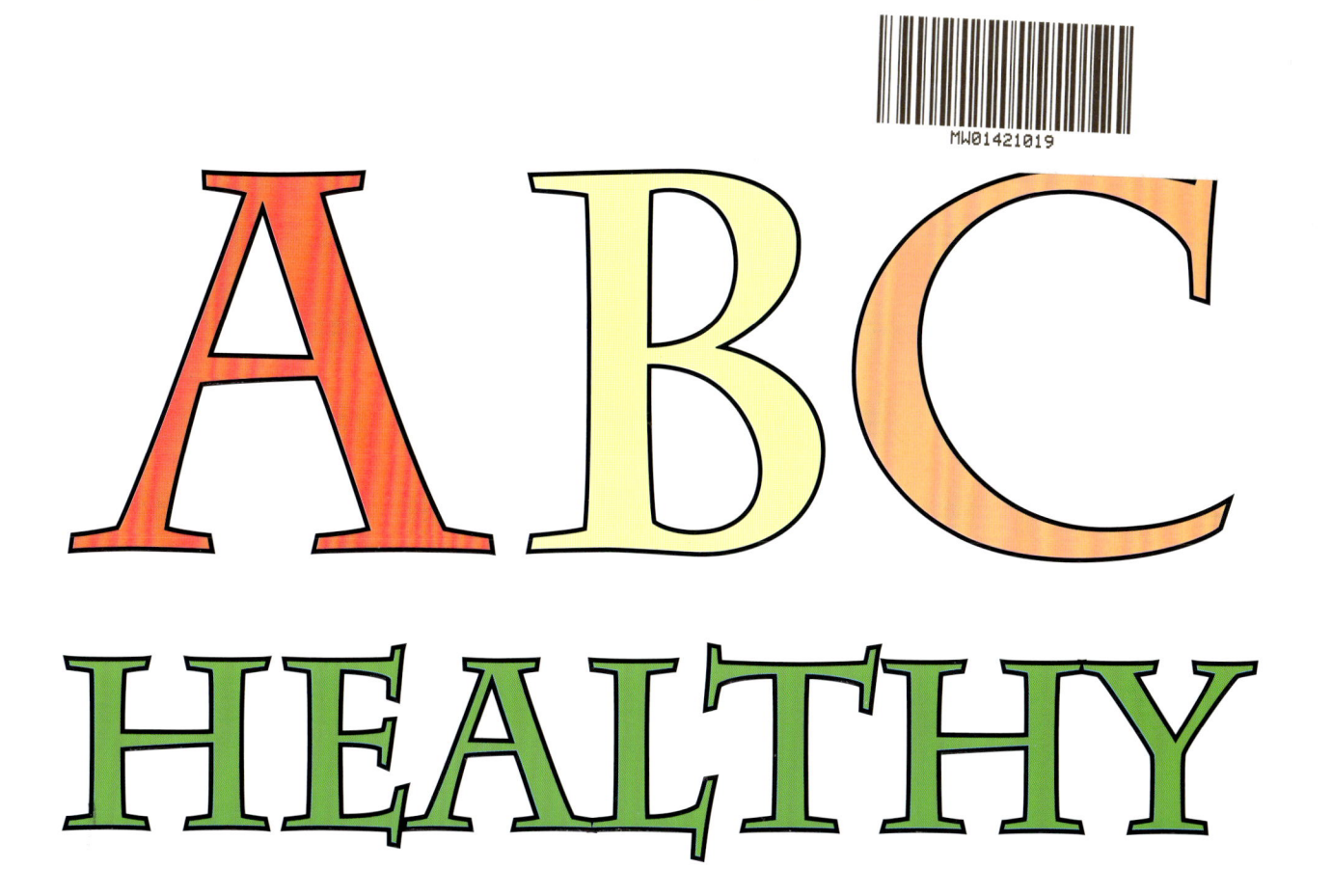

Written and Illustrated by Julianne Stokes

To Serena,
May your life be filled with health, happiness, and yummy food to eat!
♡ Julie

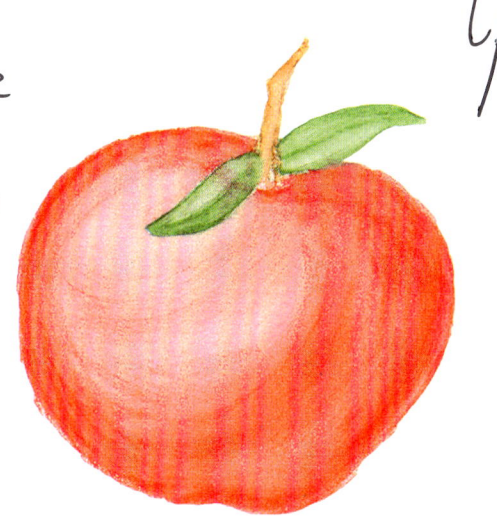

To my two boys, Jimmy and Ansel,
who love to run, play, and eat healthy all day.

A special thank you to pediatrician,
Dr. Michael Bleiman for his expertise in
reviewing *ABC Healthy*.

Copyright © 2015 [Julianne Stokes] All Rights Reserved.
Published in Snowmass Village, Colorado.
Printed in China.
ISBN: 978-0-692-40932-9
Library of Congress Control Number: 2015904445

A is for apple, an amazing healthy pick. Eat one on the go for a snack that is quick.

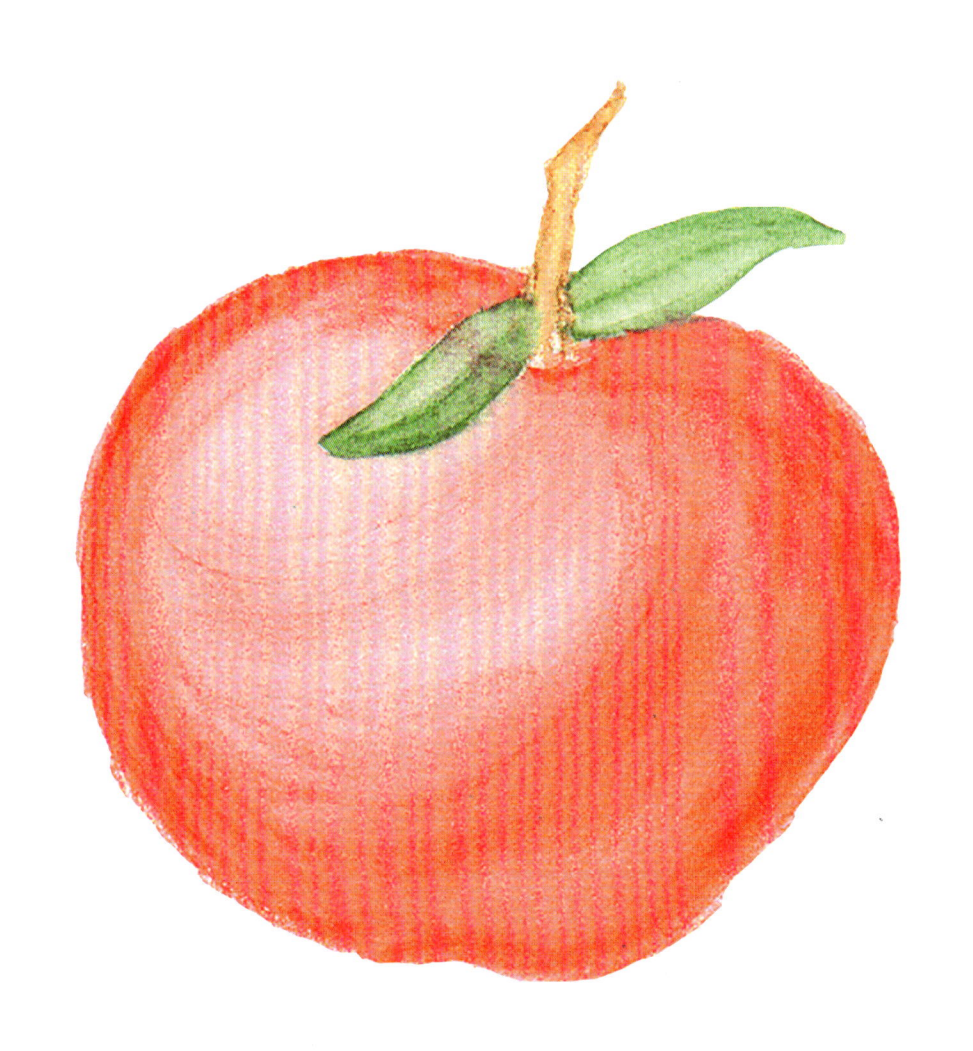

B is for banana,
best before they brown. A perfectly ripe
banana will never make you frown.

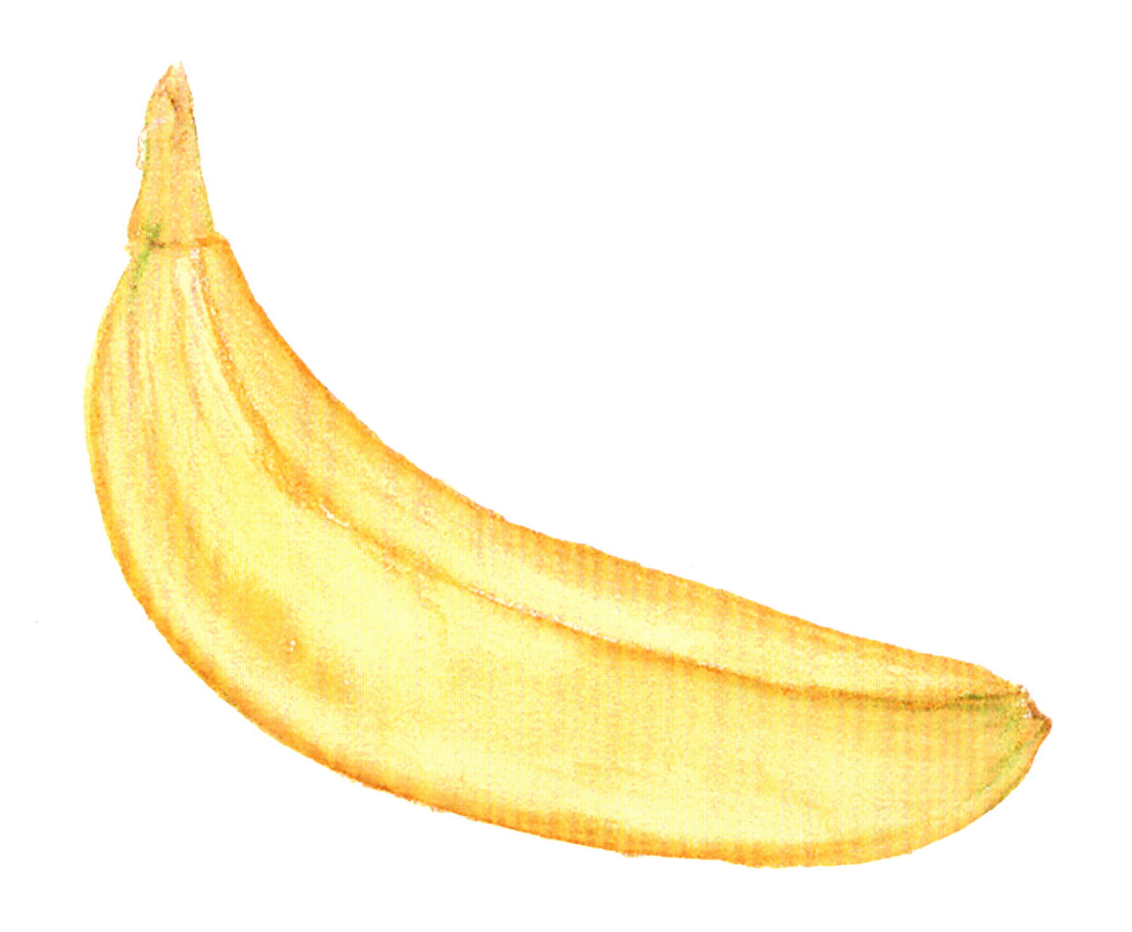

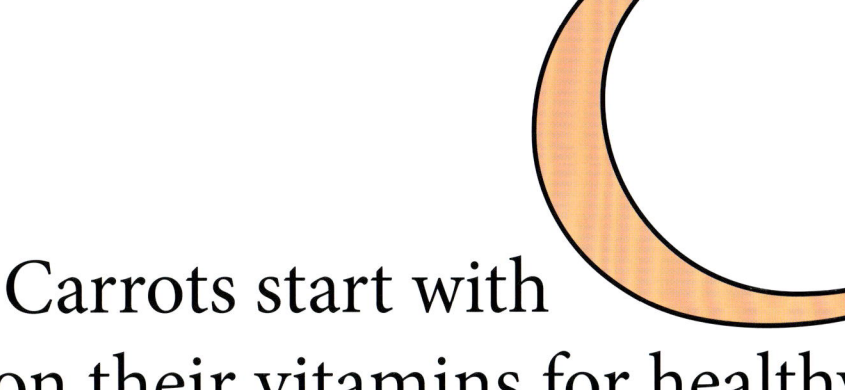

Carrots start with C
Count on their vitamins for healthy eyes.
You may not expect them to be sweet, which is a very nice surprise.

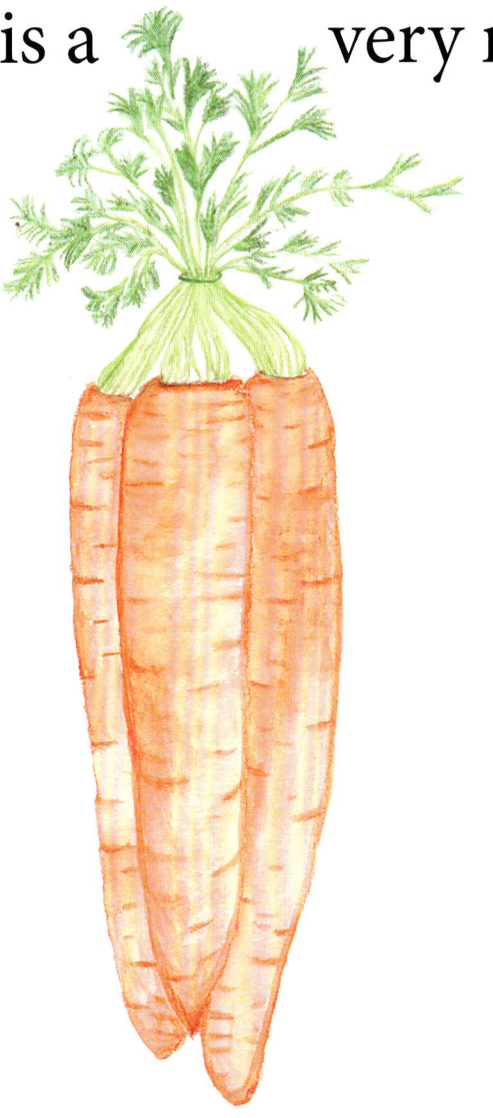

D
on't eat donuts, choose dates instead. You can eat them in the morning when you get out of bed.

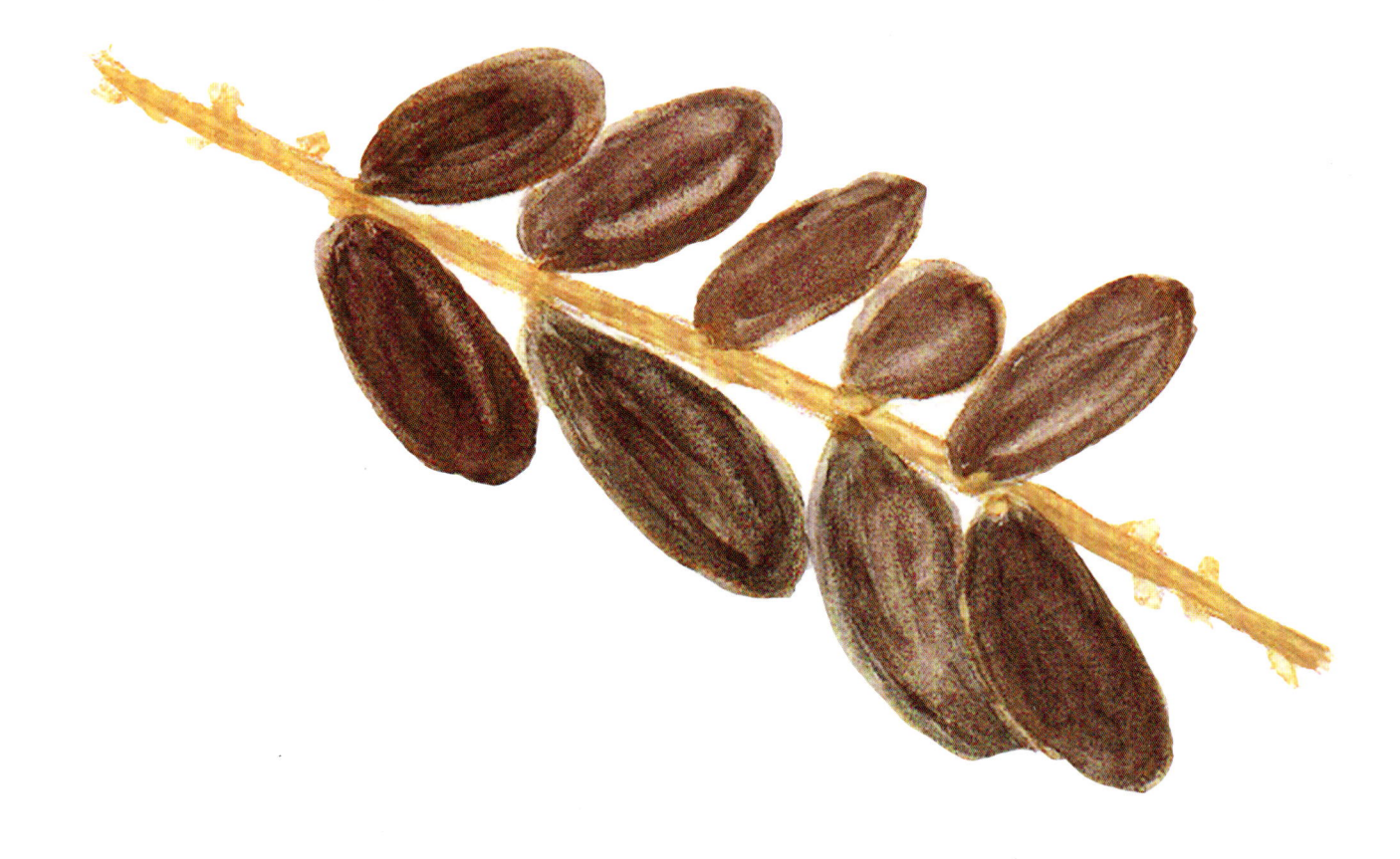

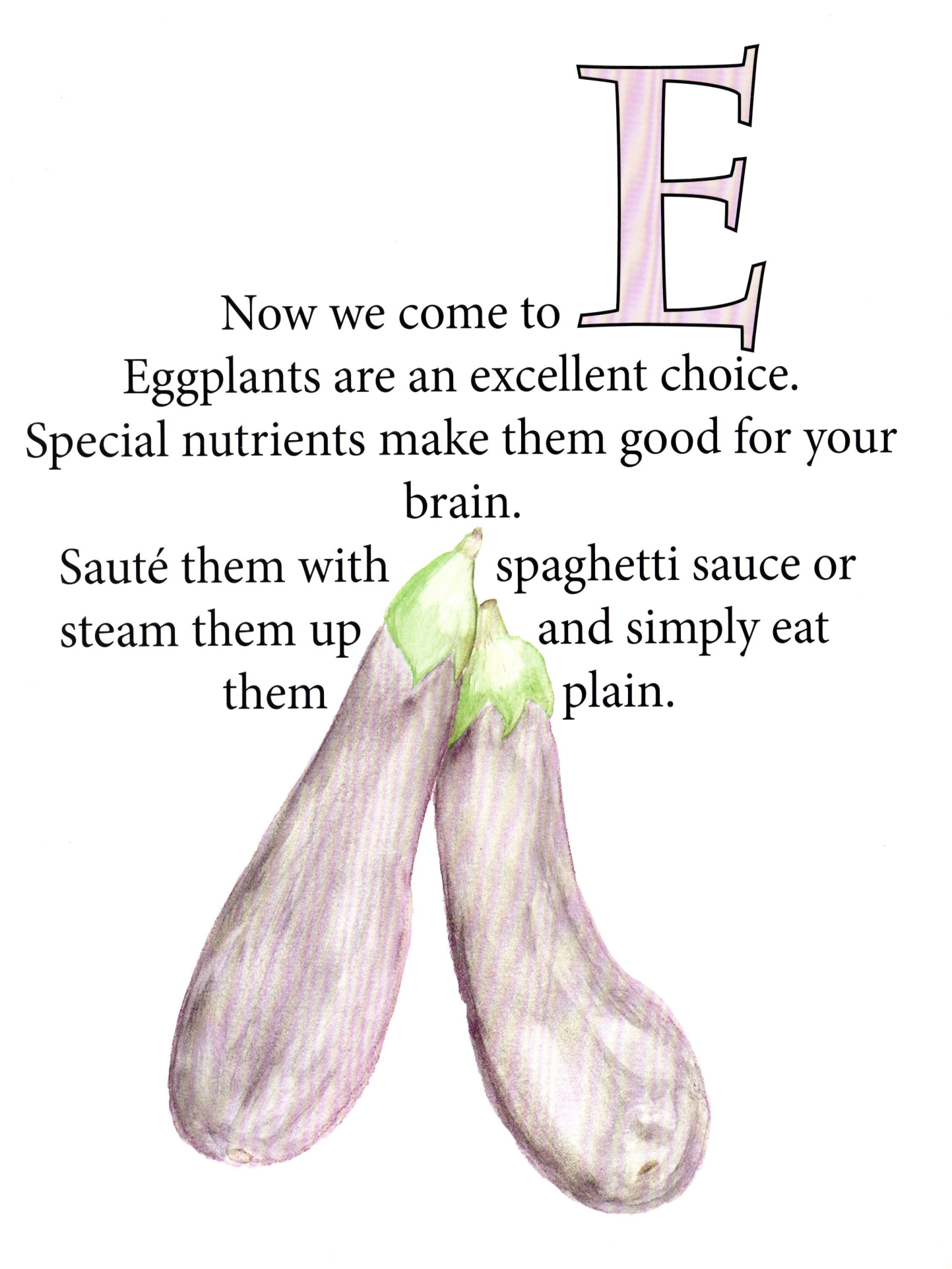

Now we come to E
Eggplants are an excellent choice.
Special nutrients make them good for your brain.
Sauté them with spaghetti sauce or steam them up and simply eat them plain.

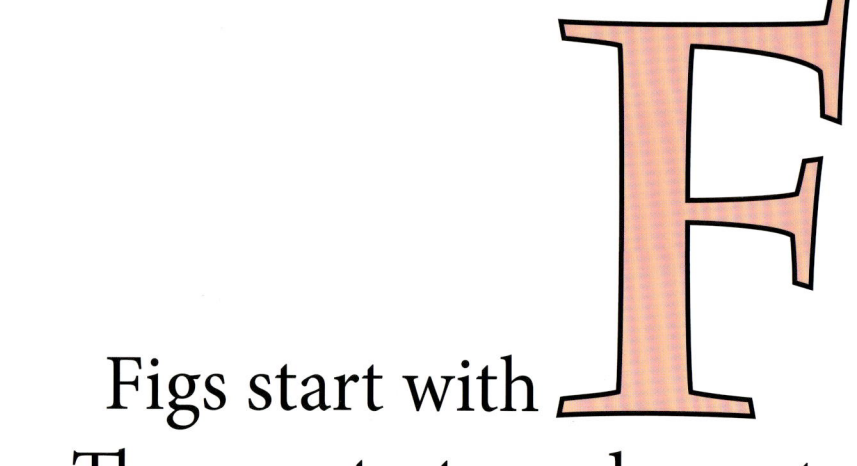

Figs start with F
They are tasty and sweet.
Eating them will be a very special treat.

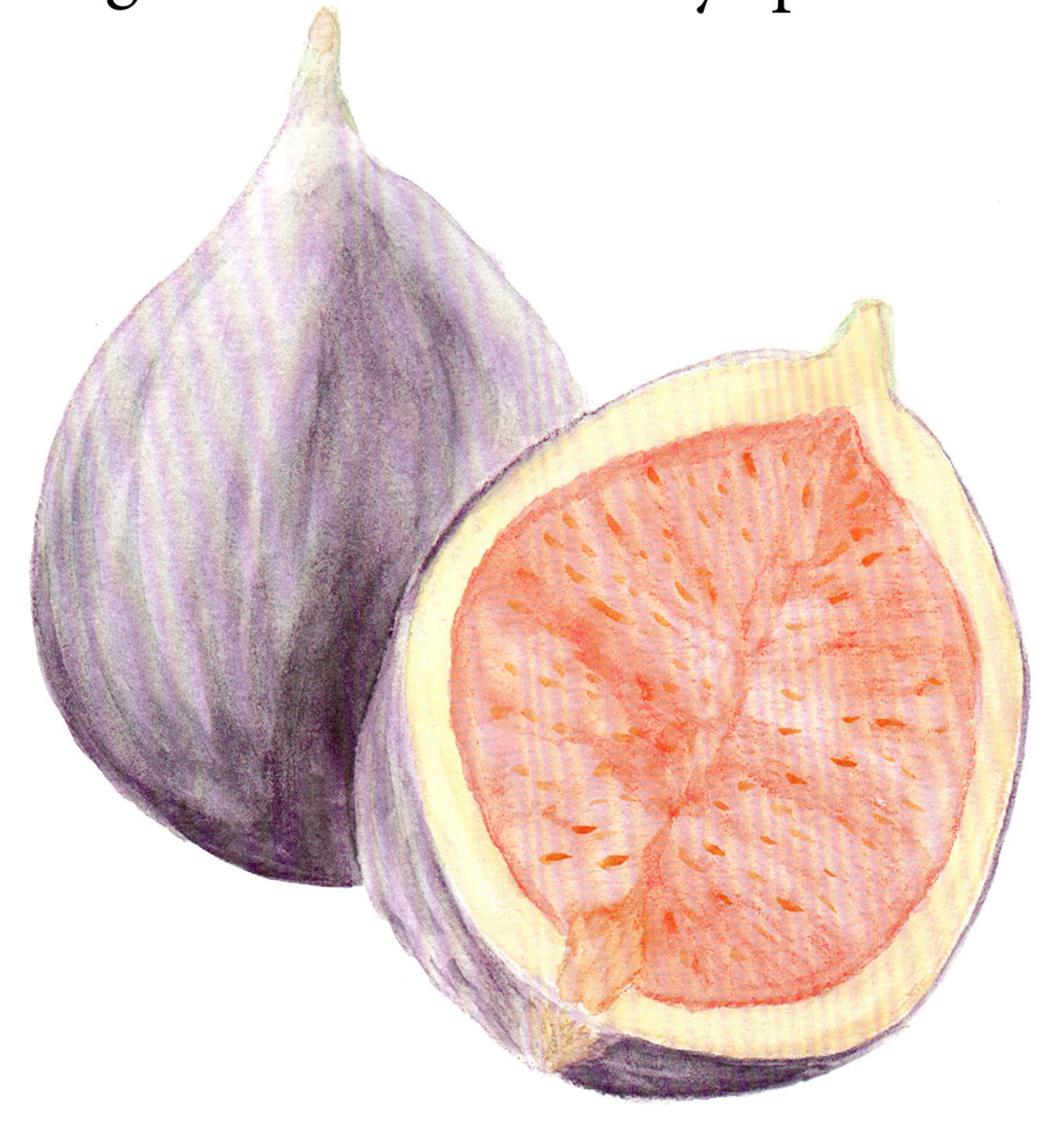

G is for grapes. Grapes are filled with the nutrients to help your body keep well. Not only are they good for you, but they sure taste swell.

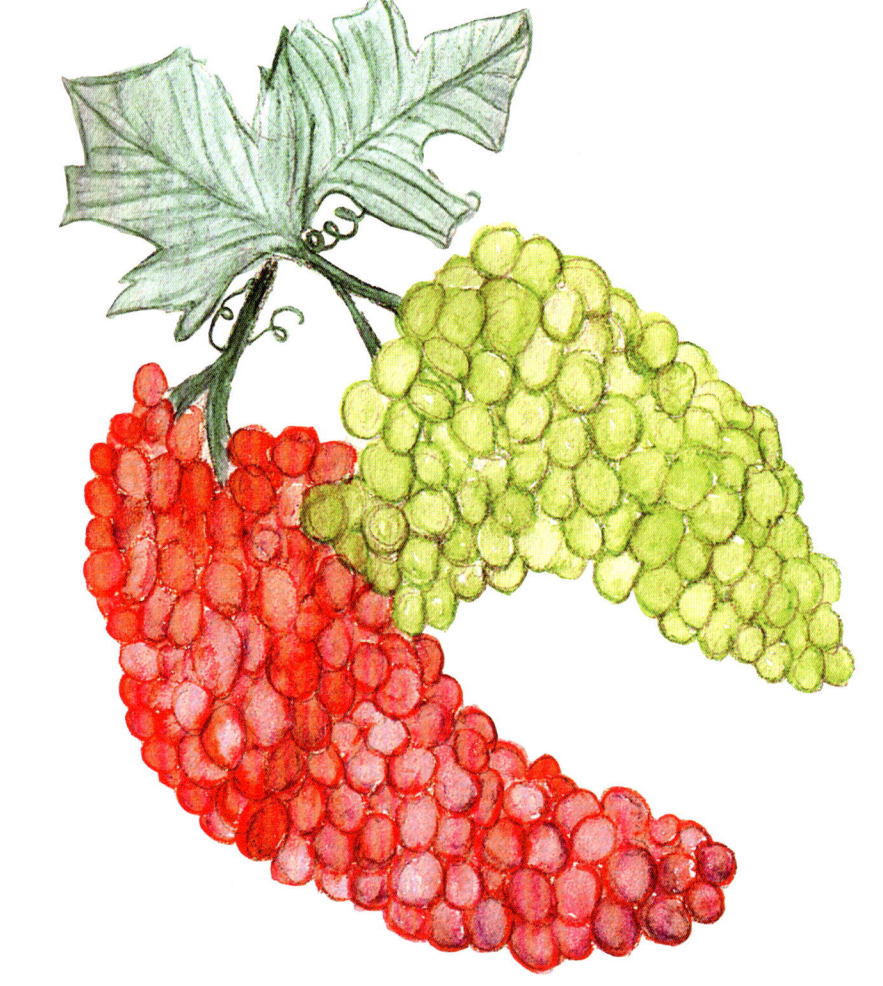

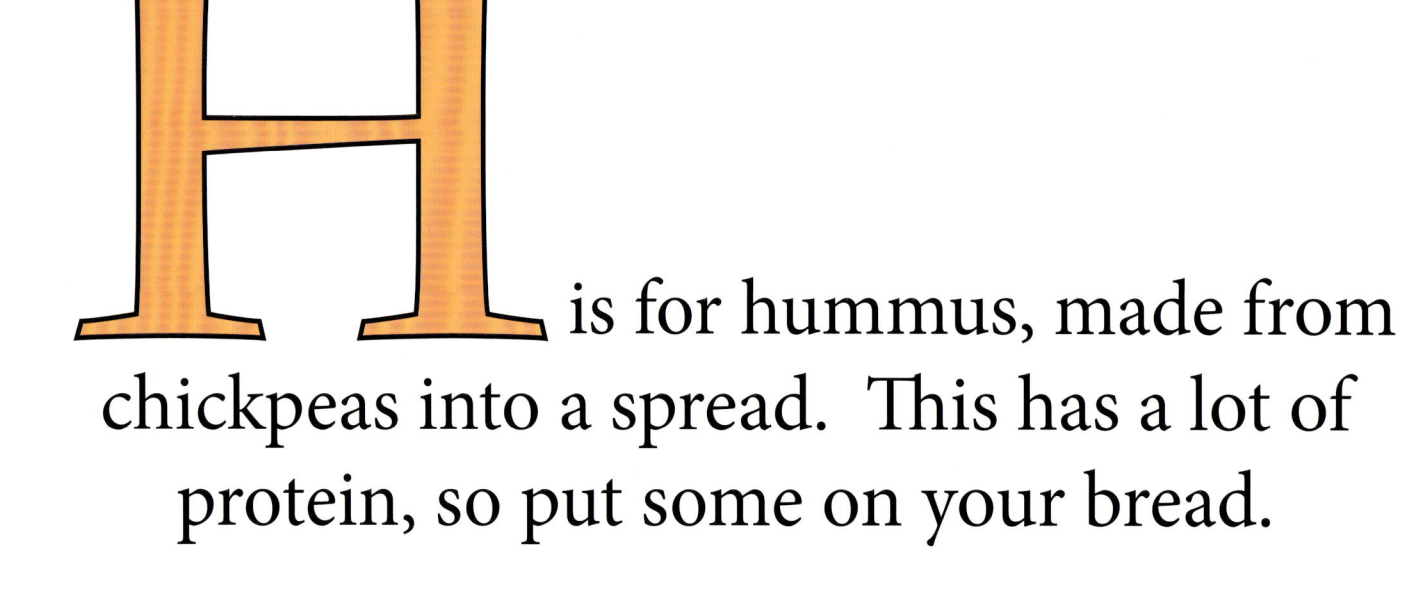

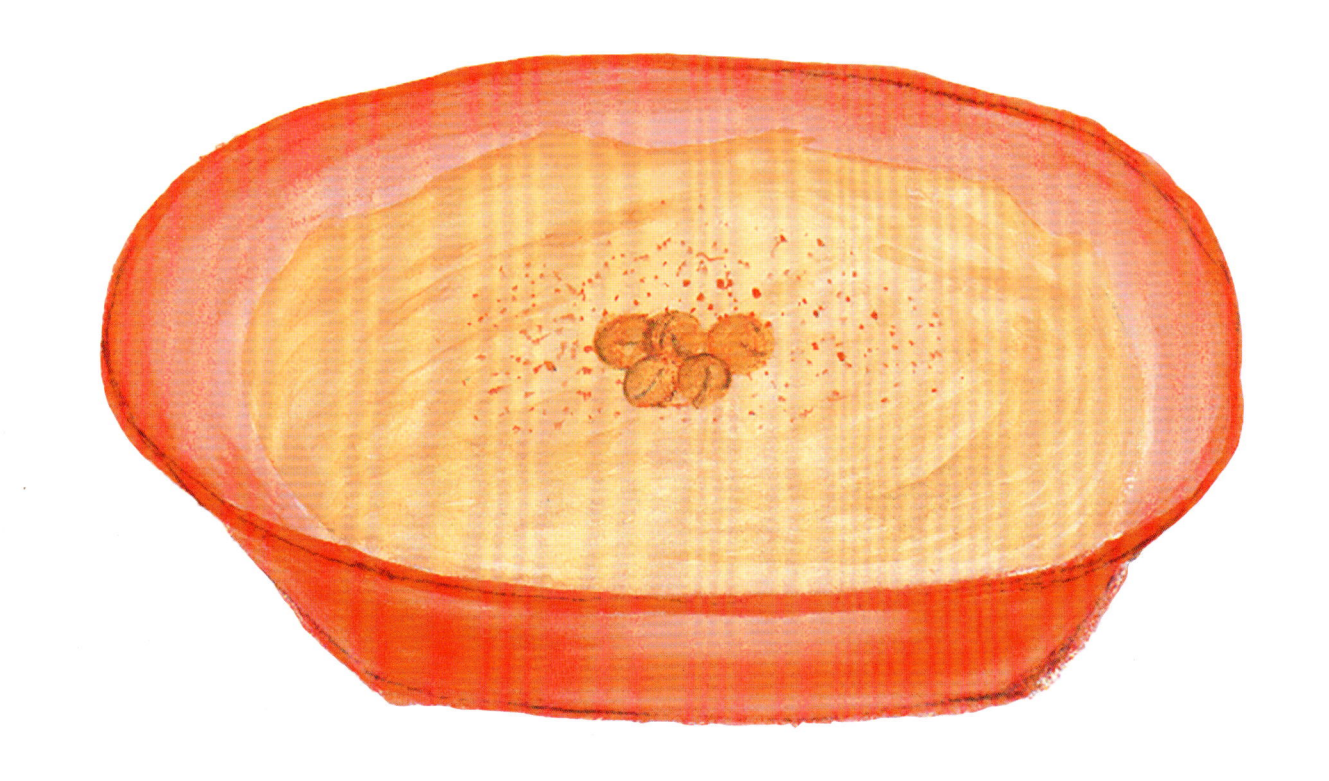

H is for hummus, made from chickpeas into a spread. This has a lot of protein, so put some on your bread.

I is for ice to keep your water cold.
Water will make you feel strong and bold.

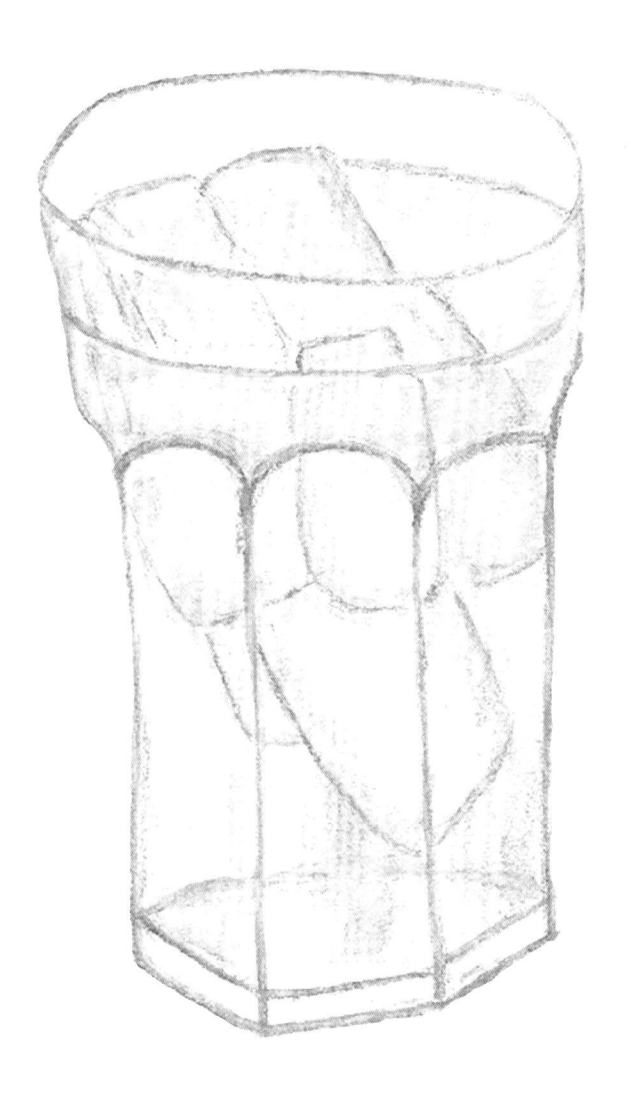

J is for juice, good in small amounts. Enjoy it with some pulp and make the fiber count.

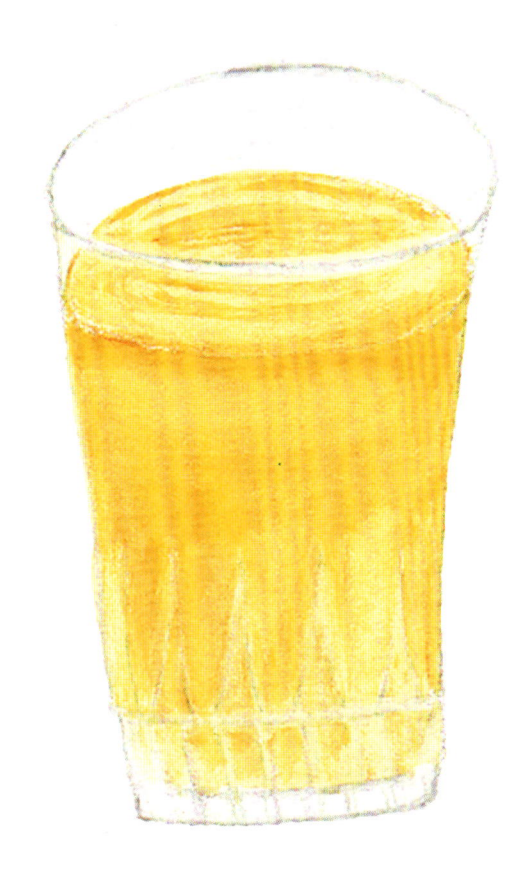

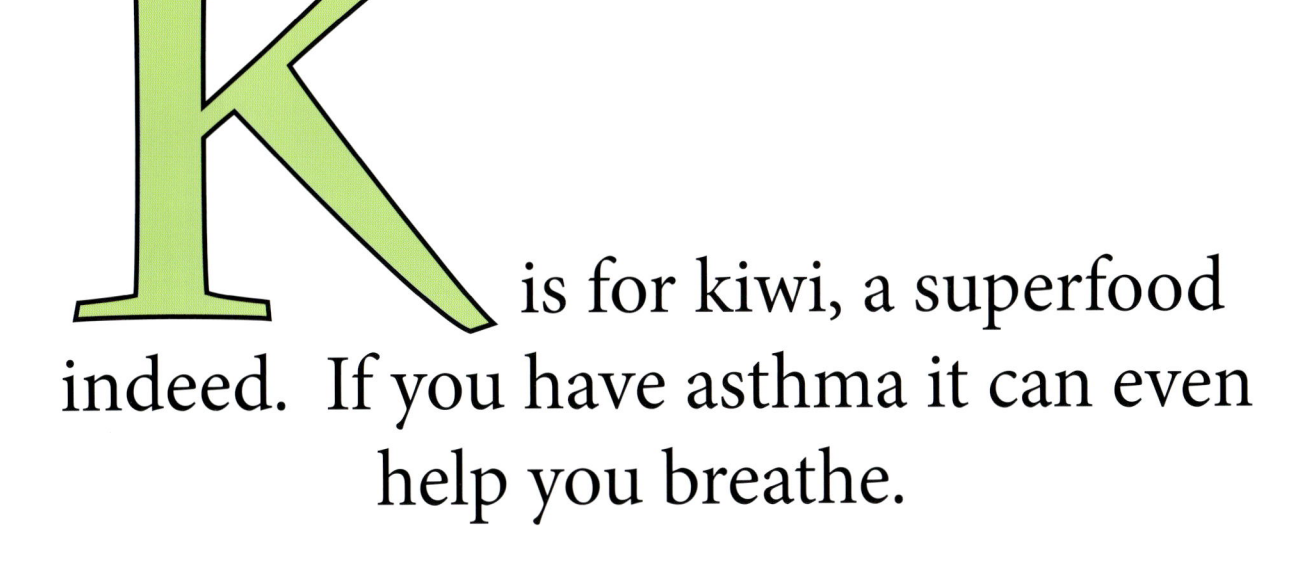

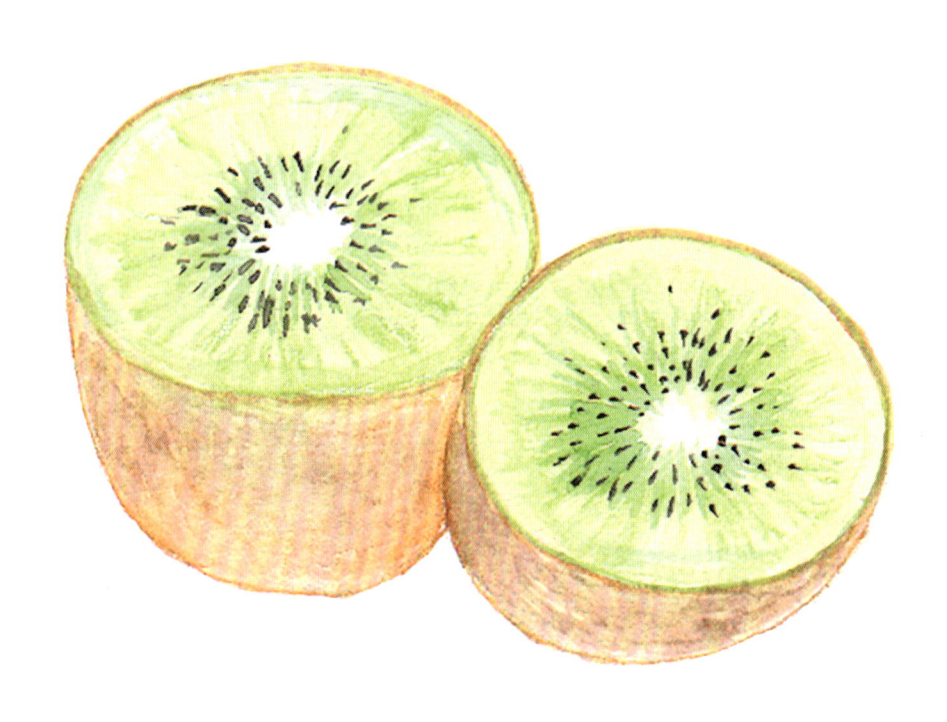

K is for kiwi, a superfood indeed. If you have asthma it can even help you breathe.

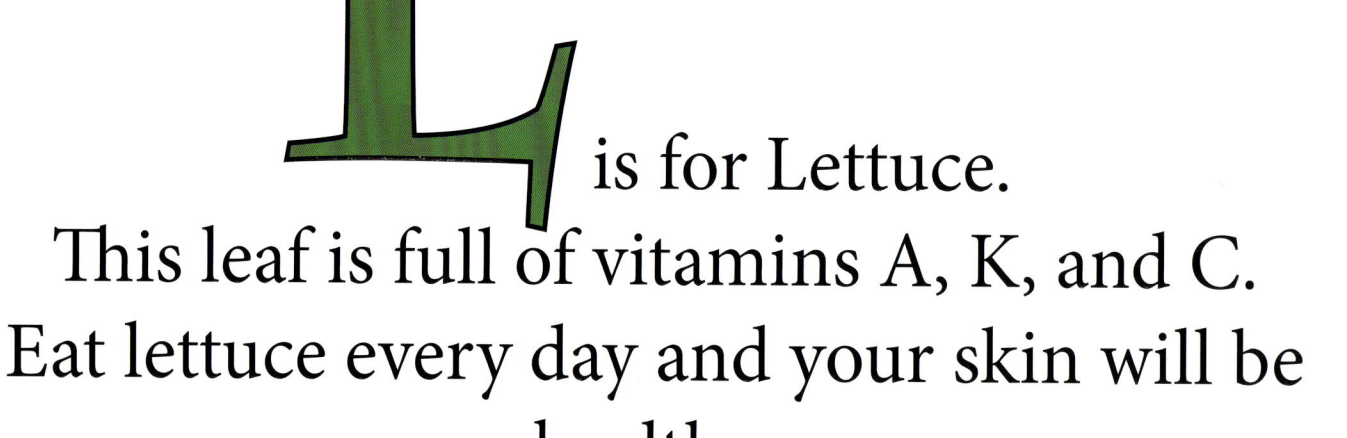

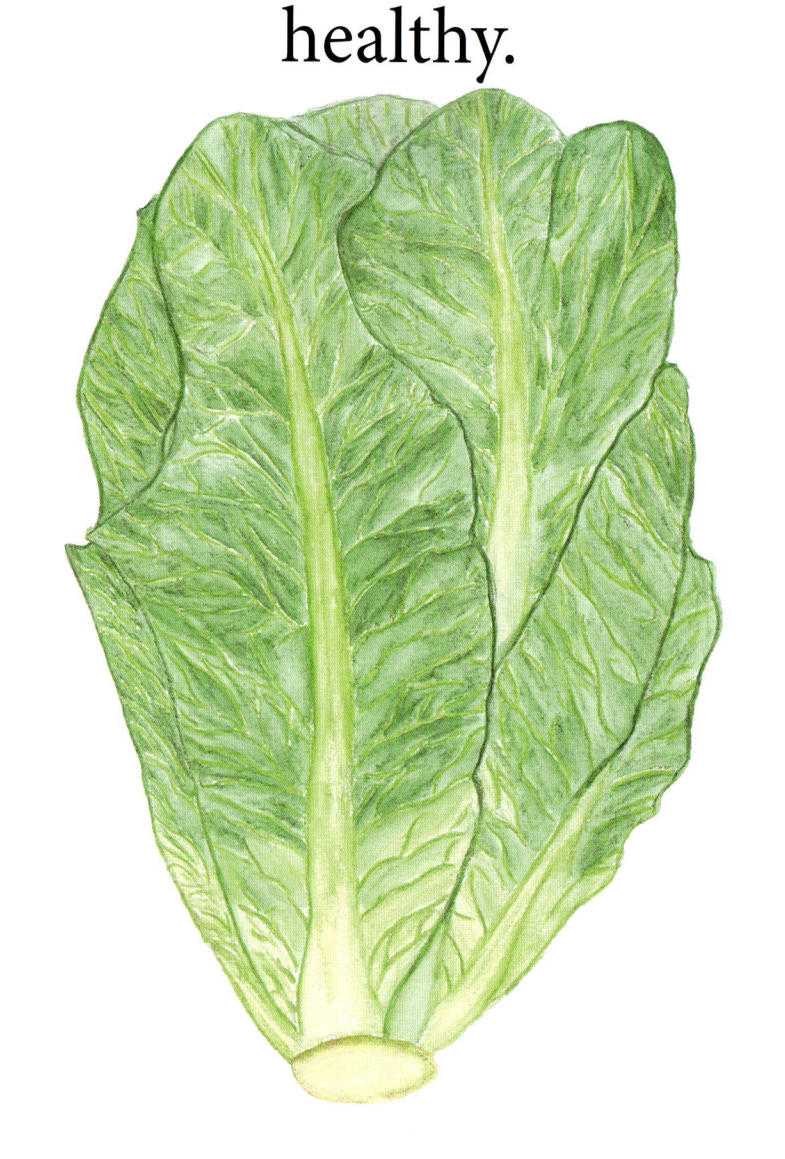

L is for Lettuce.
This leaf is full of vitamins A, K, and C. Eat lettuce every day and your skin will be healthy.

M is for mushrooms. You can eat them raw or cooked. They are so rich and yummy your taste buds will be hooked.

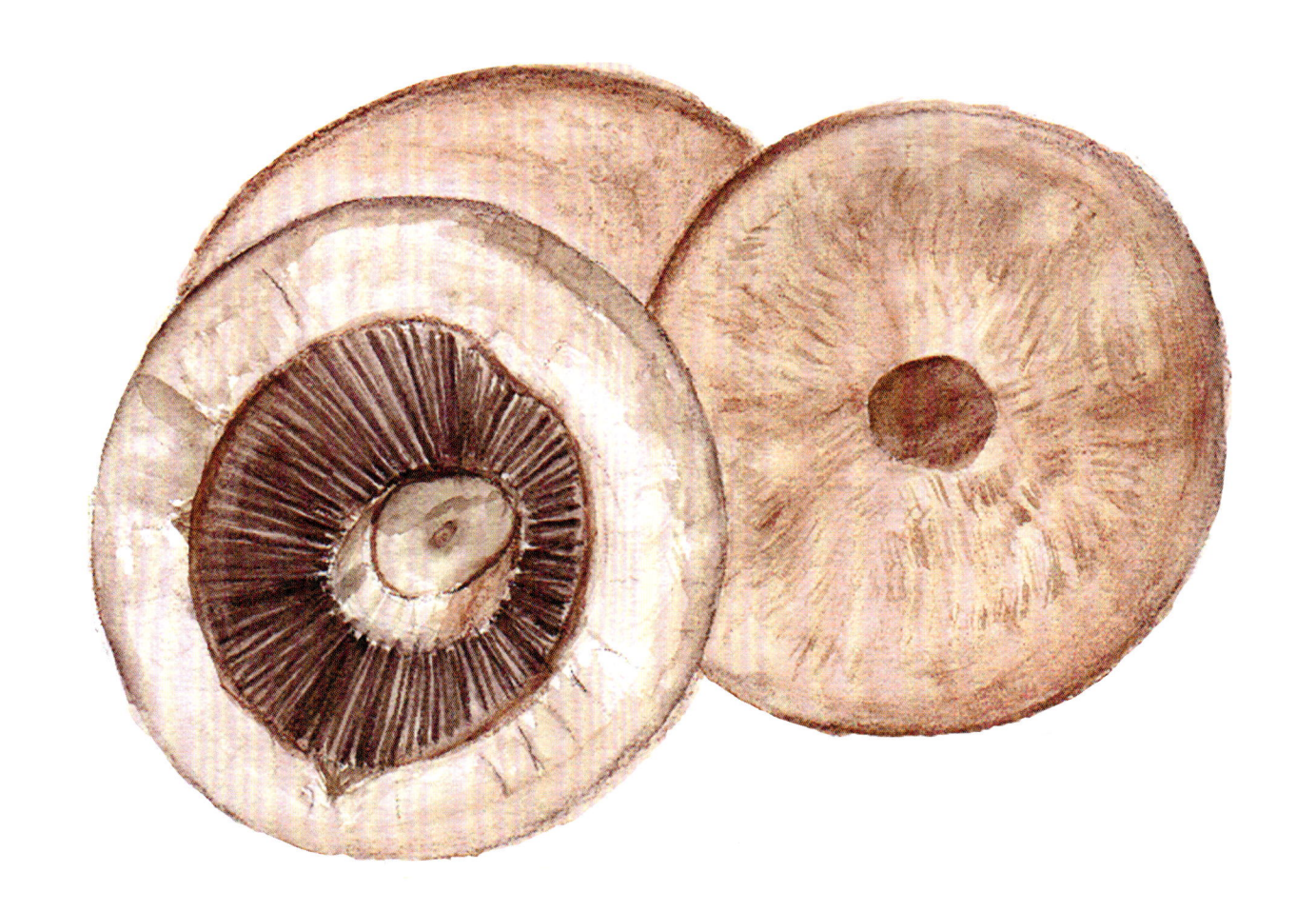

Never leave the house without nuts.

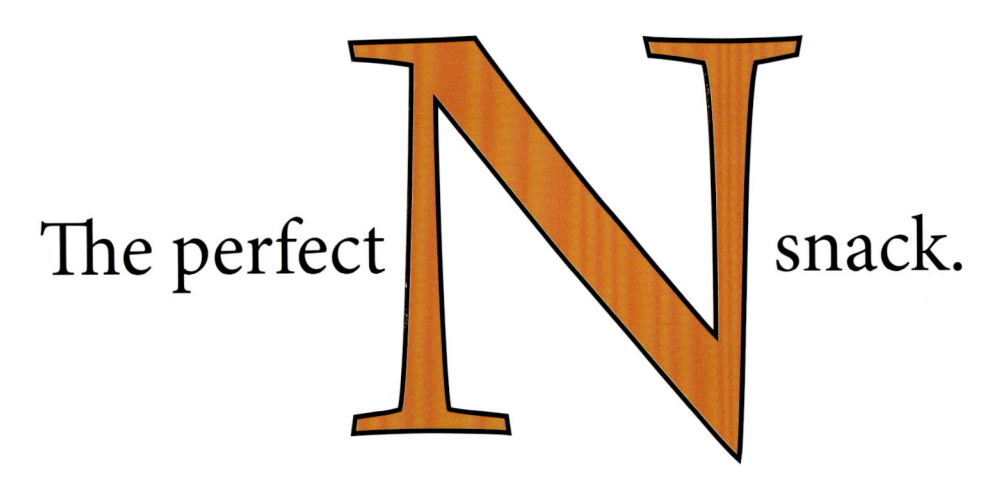

N

The perfect N snack.

They are filled with
fiber, protein, and healthy fats!

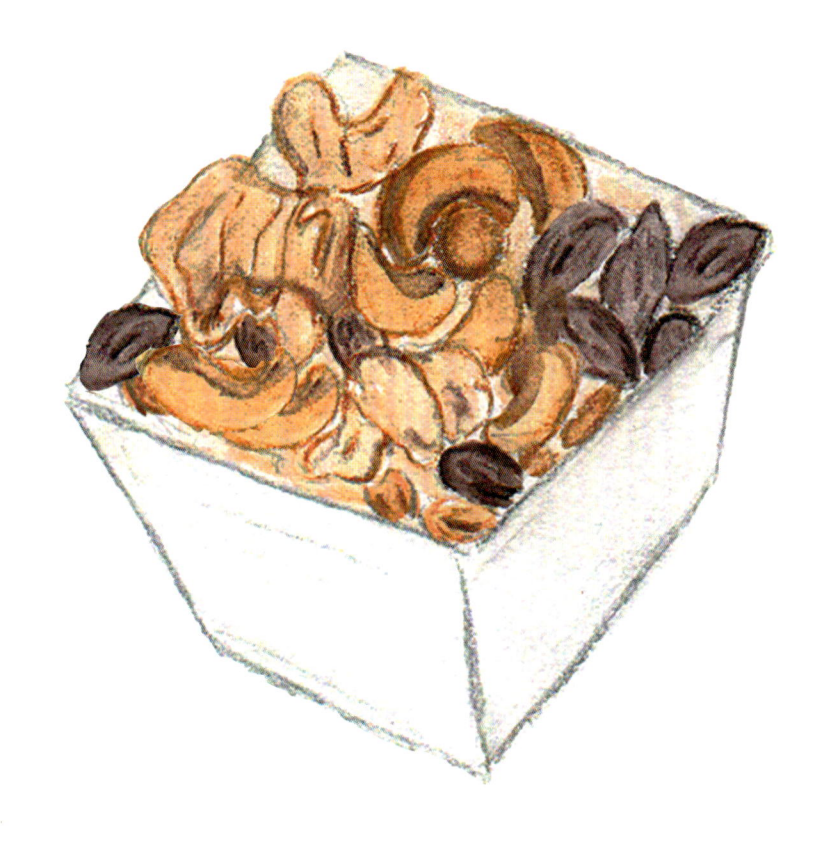

O is for orange, the color that is true. Did you know that it is healthy to eat different colored fruits, too?

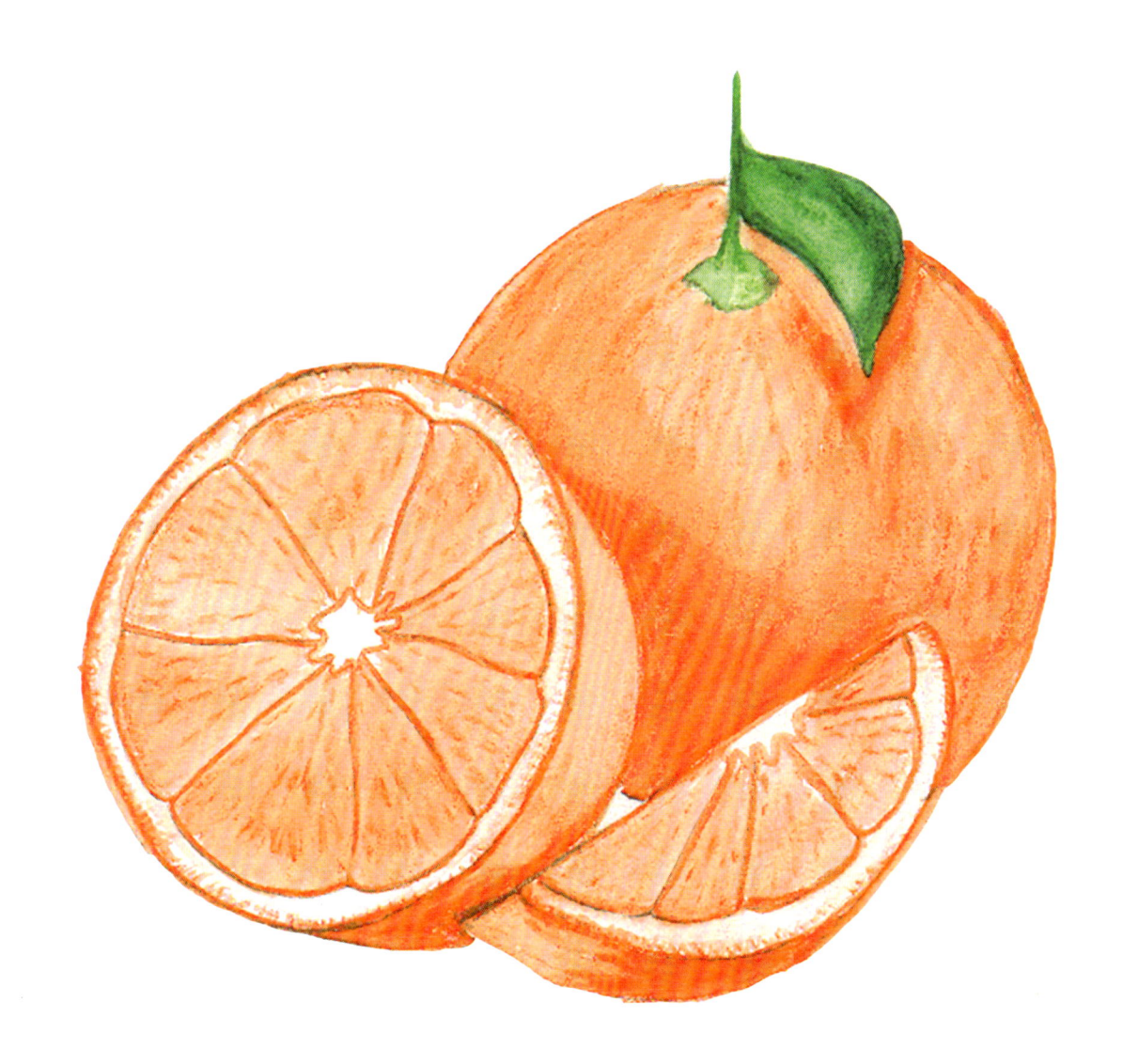

Here are some **P** foods. You will find more colors here: pumpkin, plum, peach, and pomegranate too. Pick some peppers and eat them until you are through.

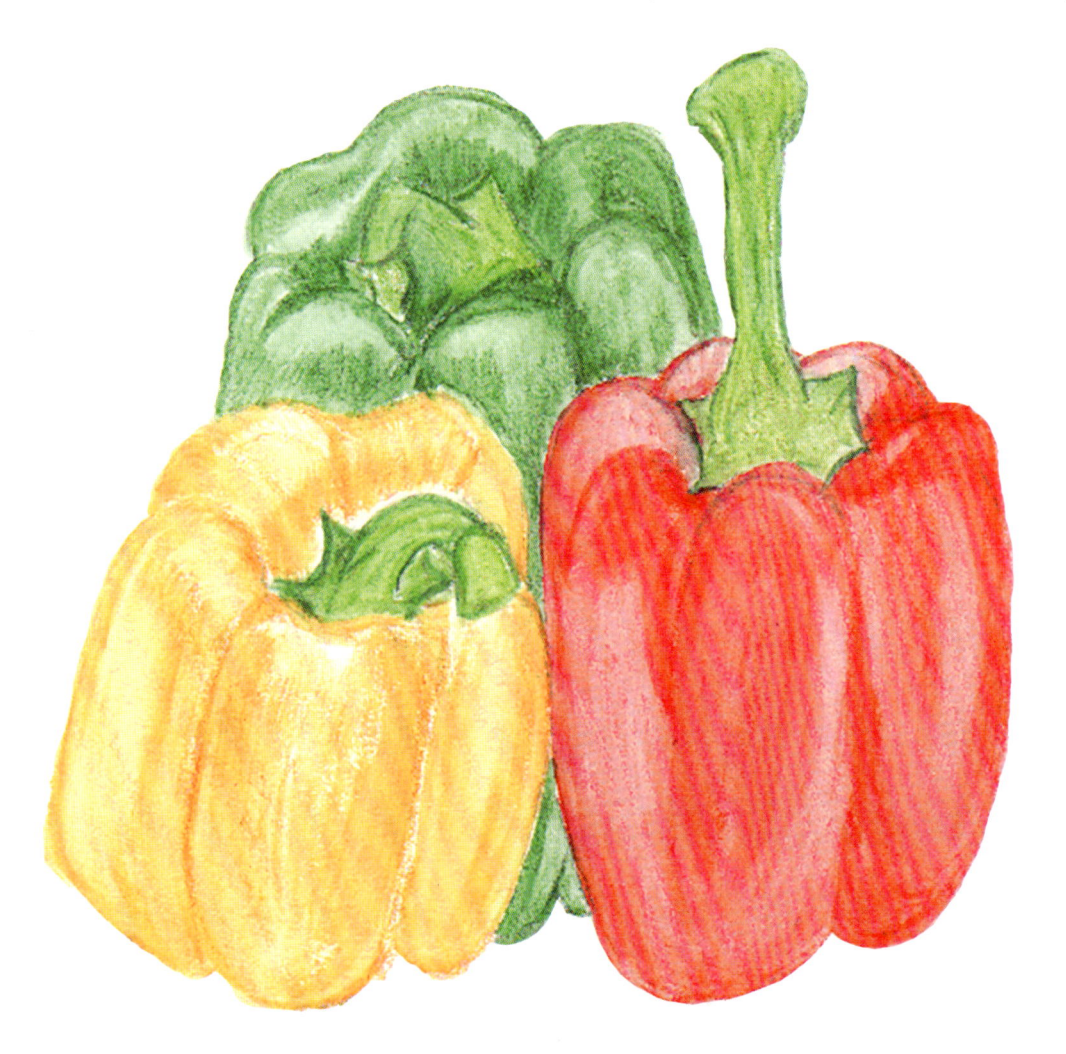

Quinoa sounds quite mysterious.

Is that because it starts with Q

This carbohydrate is filled with fiber, phosphorous, magnesium, and iron for you.

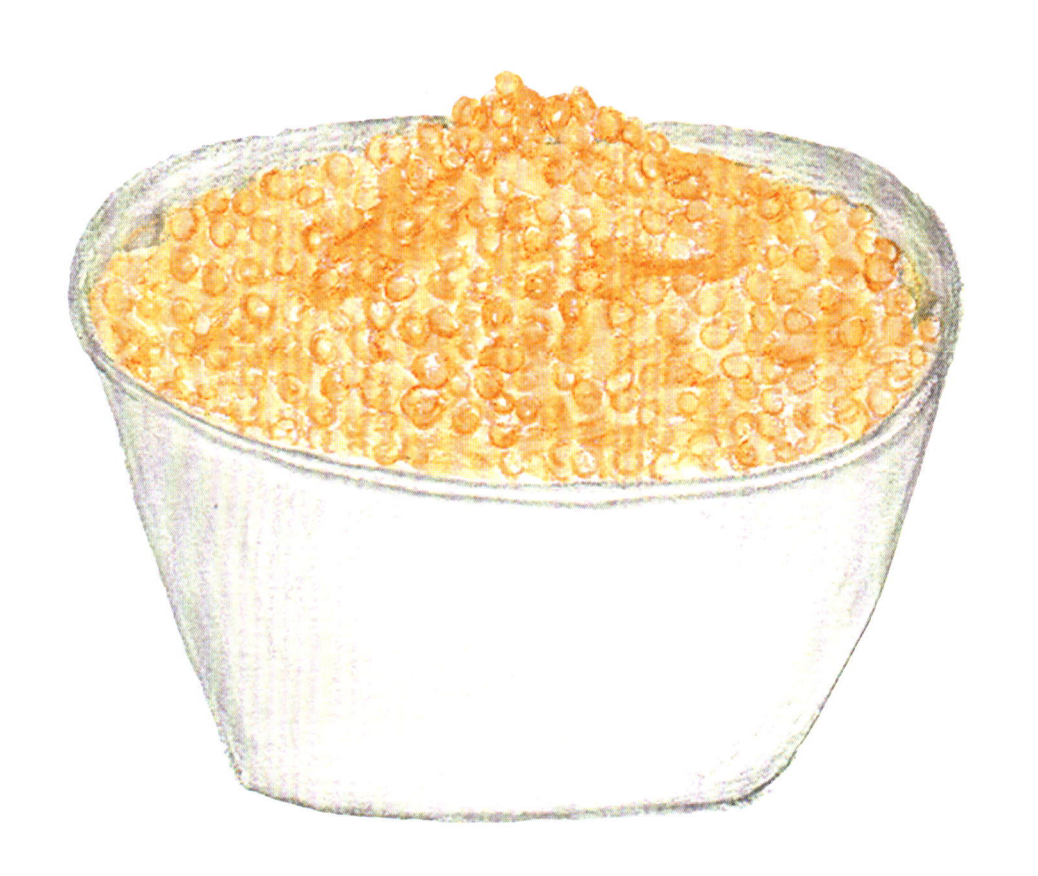

R is for red radishes, ready from the ground. Slice them up or eat them full and round.

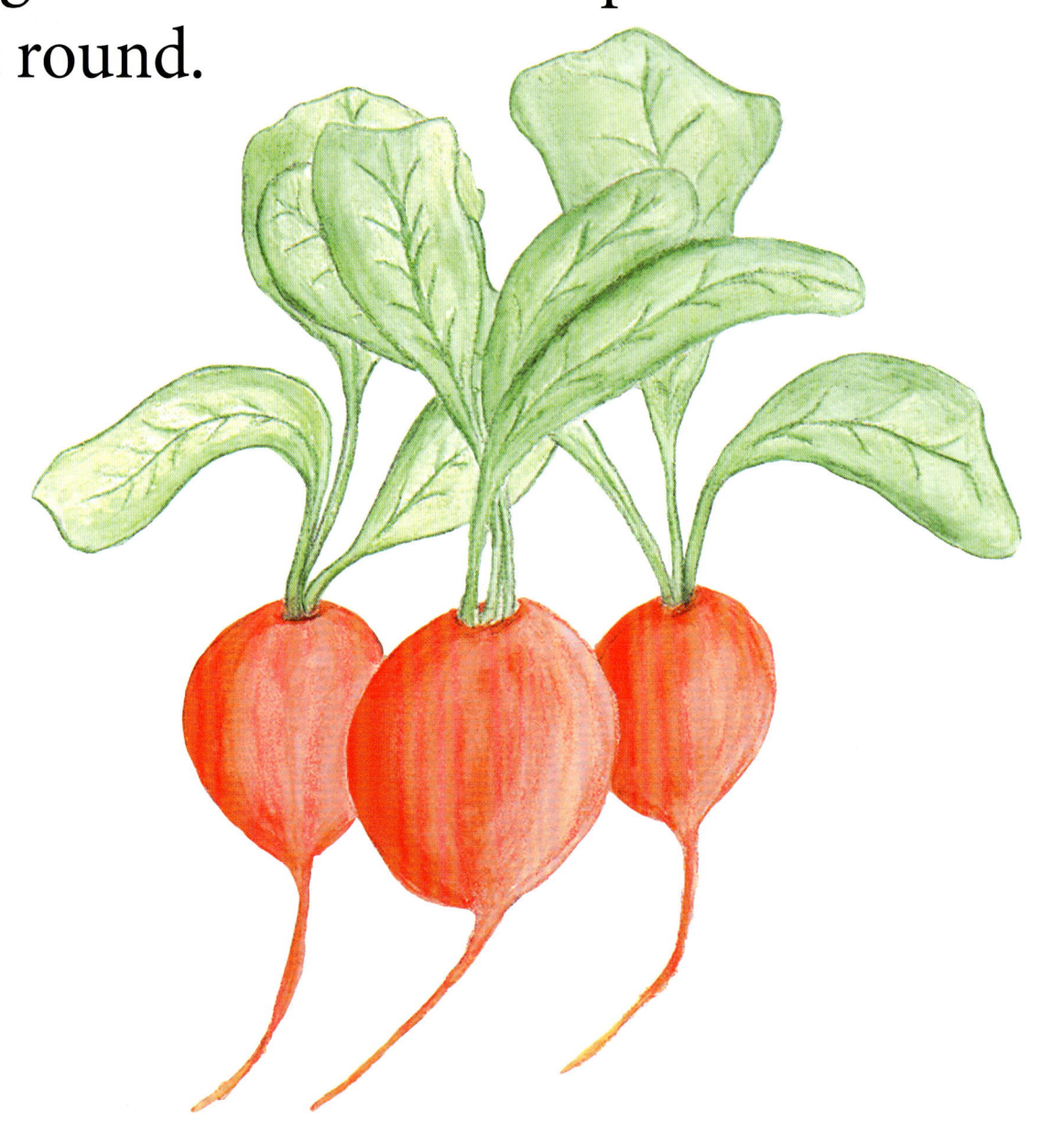

S is for spinach, a savory dark green leaf. There are so many vitamins and minerals you would be in disbelief.

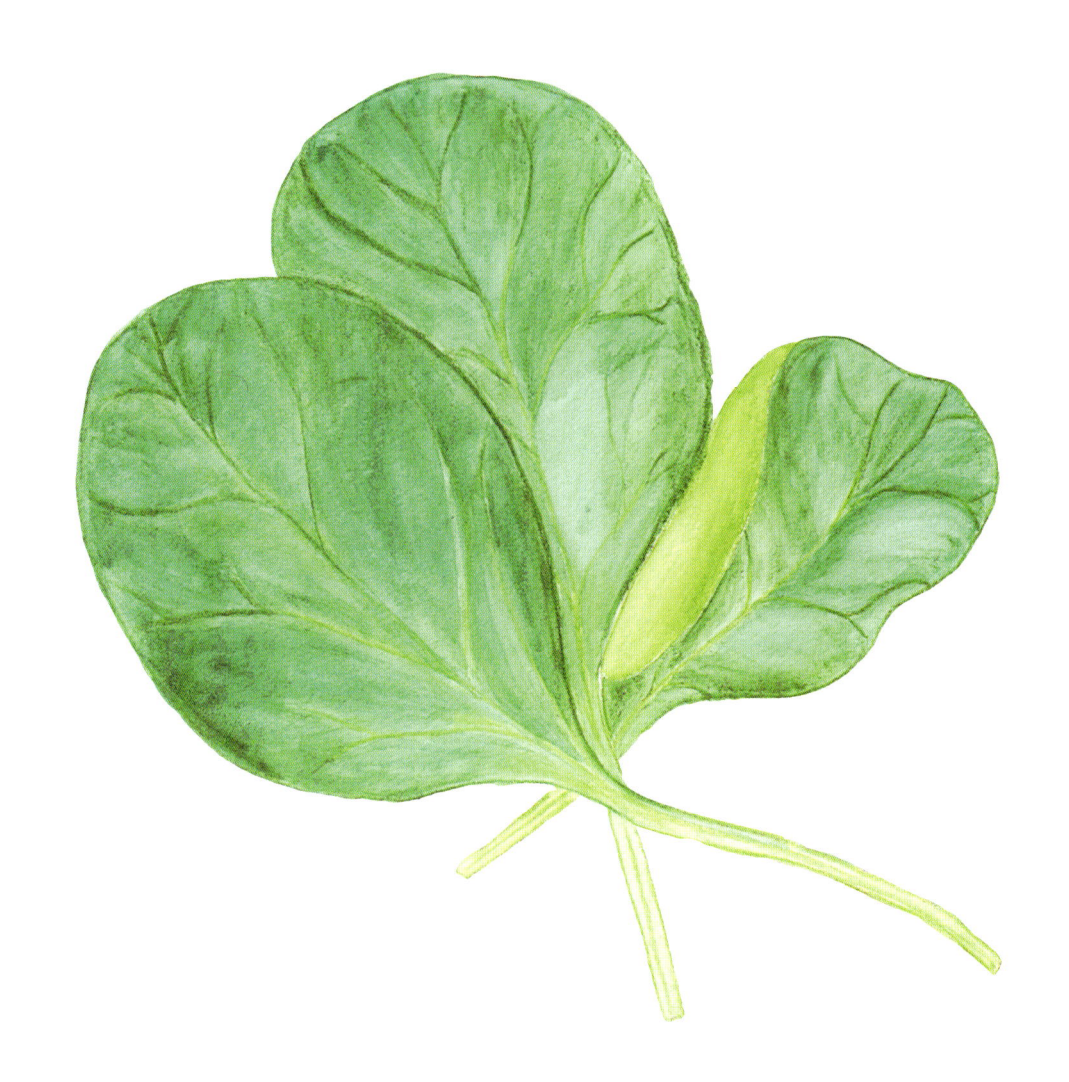

T is for tomatoes, red, juicy, and round. They are so delicious you will want to eat them by the pound.

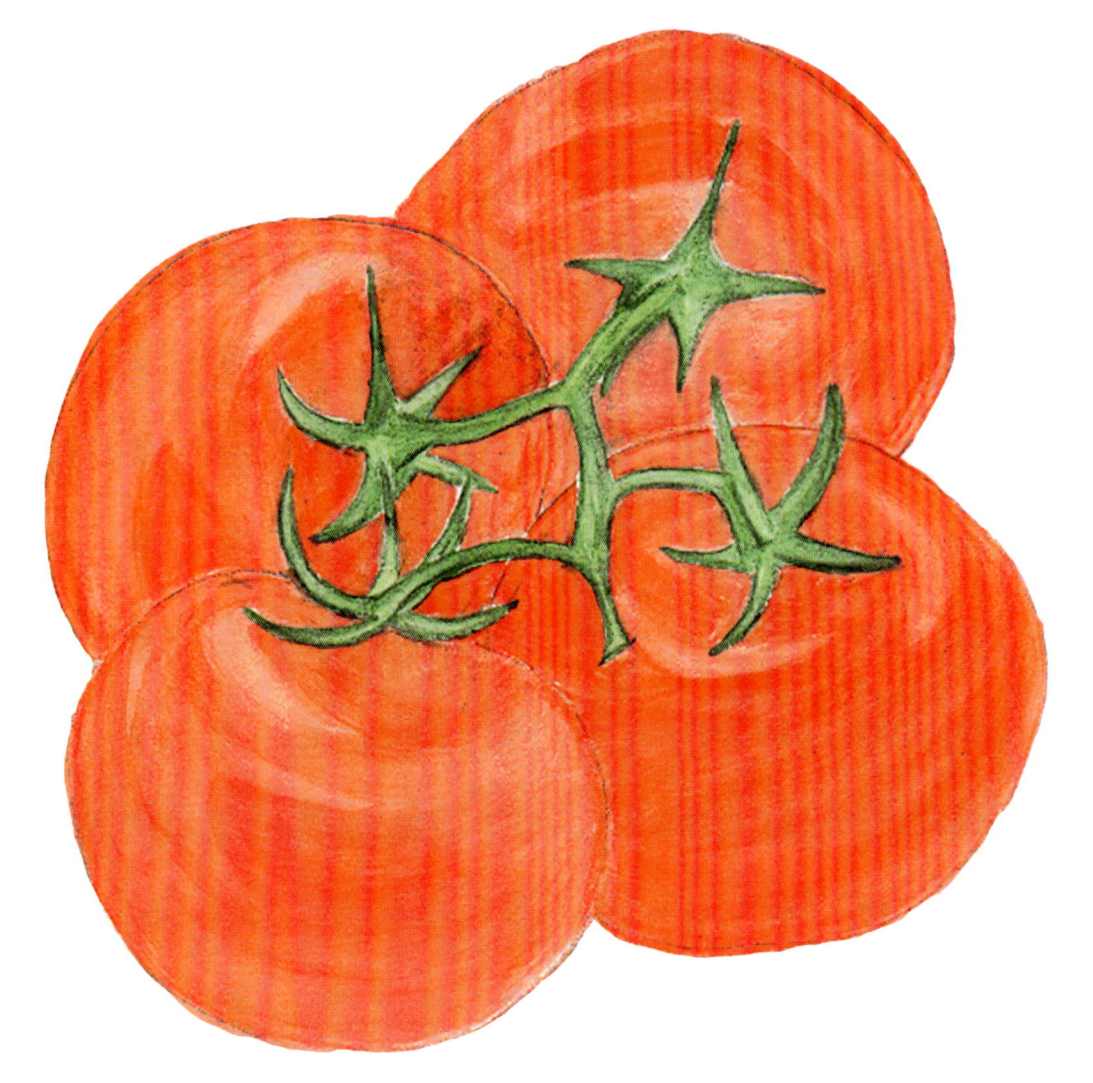

U

U is for ugli fruit, filled with fiber and vitamin C. If you can't find it in a store grab a tangerine.

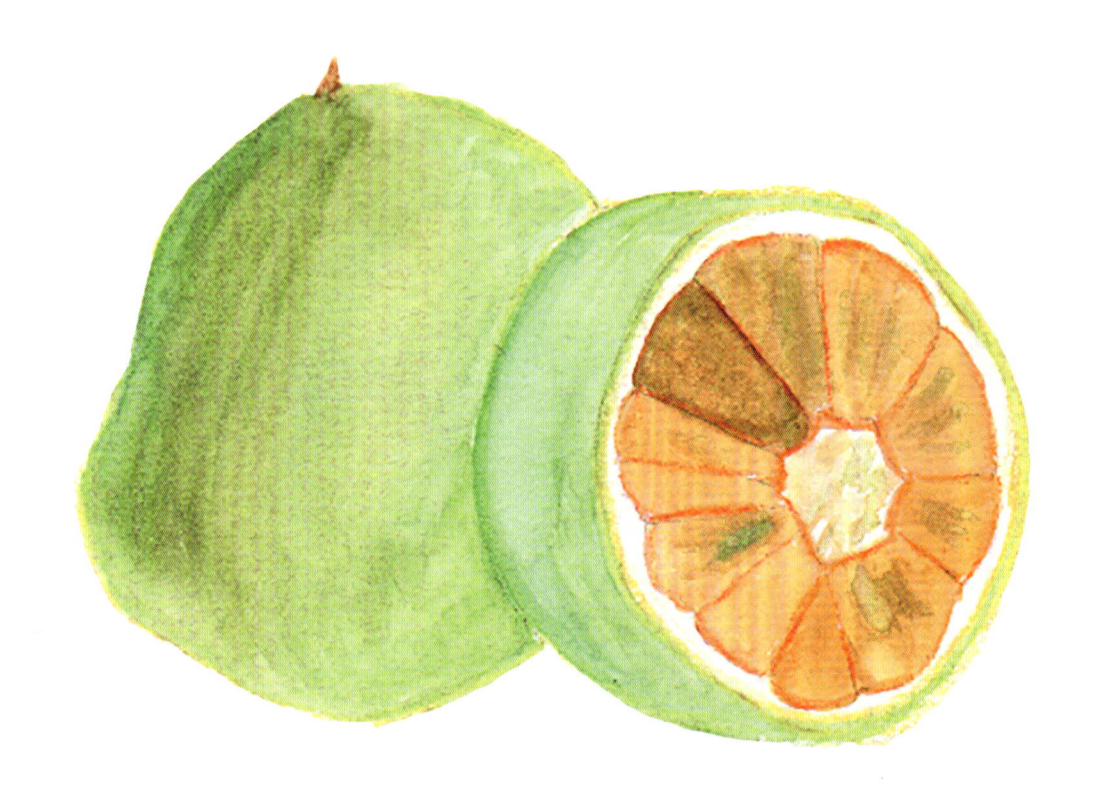

V

Victoria plum starts with V
This is another tricky find. All plums are filled with the nutritional power to help your body unwind.

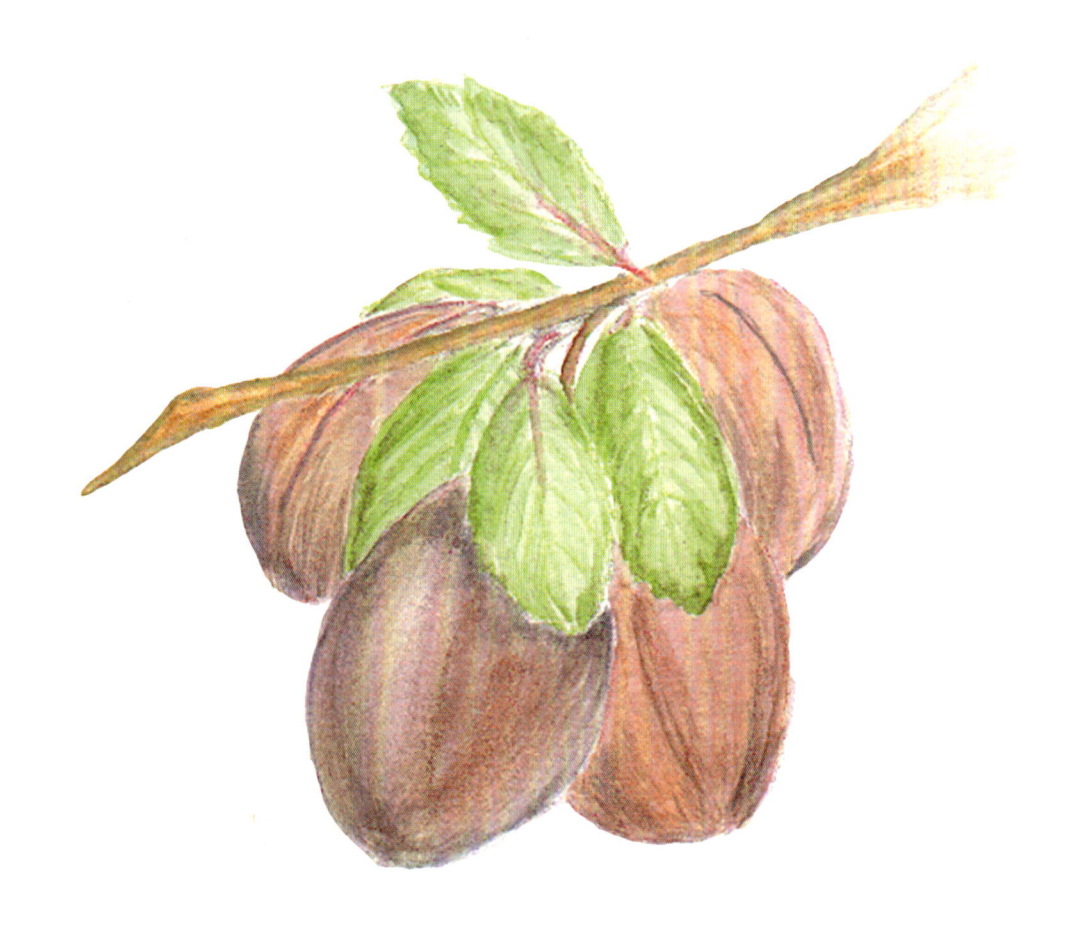

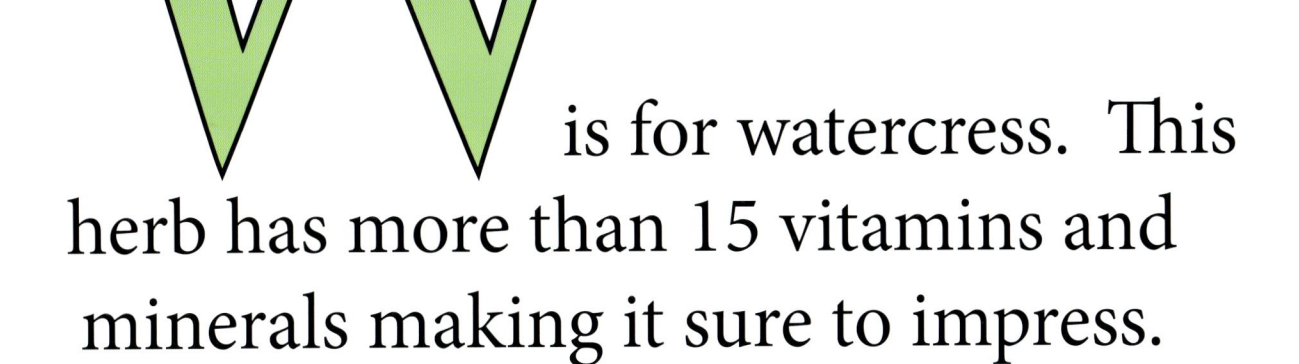

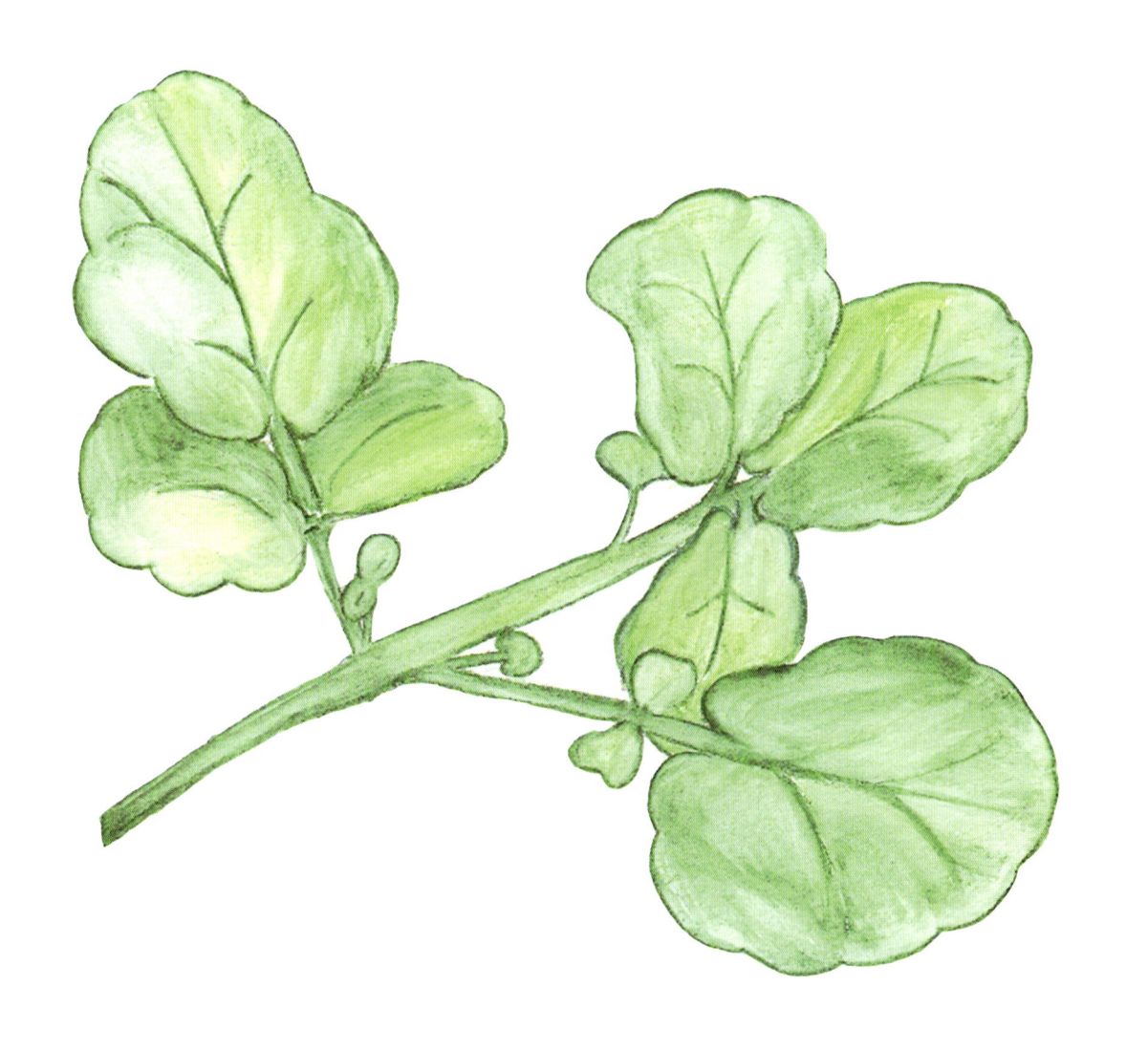

W is for watercress. This herb has more than 15 vitamins and minerals making it sure to impress.

X is for xigua (shi-gwah), another name for watermelon. There are many types of this excellent fruit. It is so juicy it will make you holler and hoot.

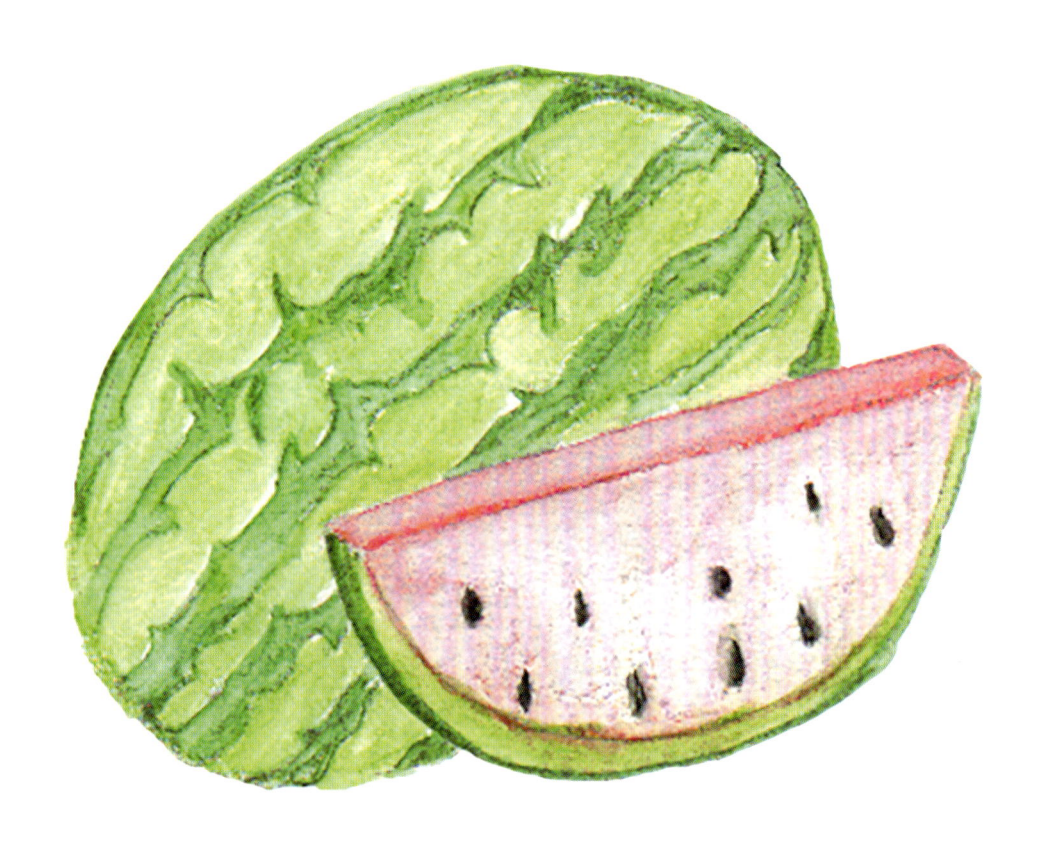

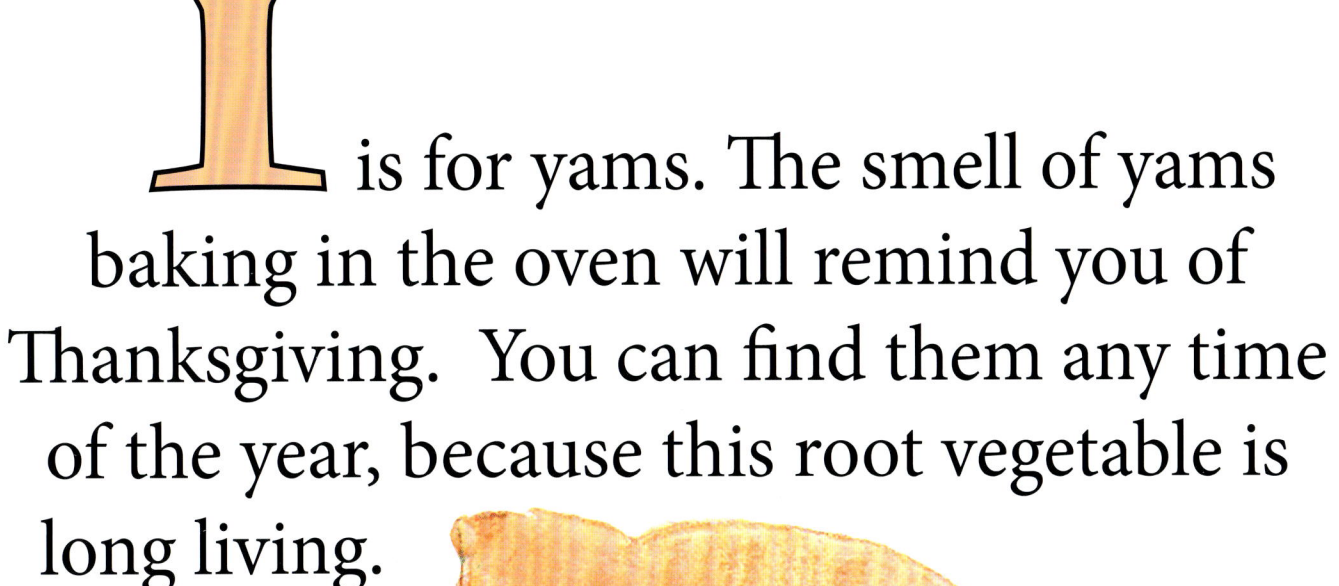

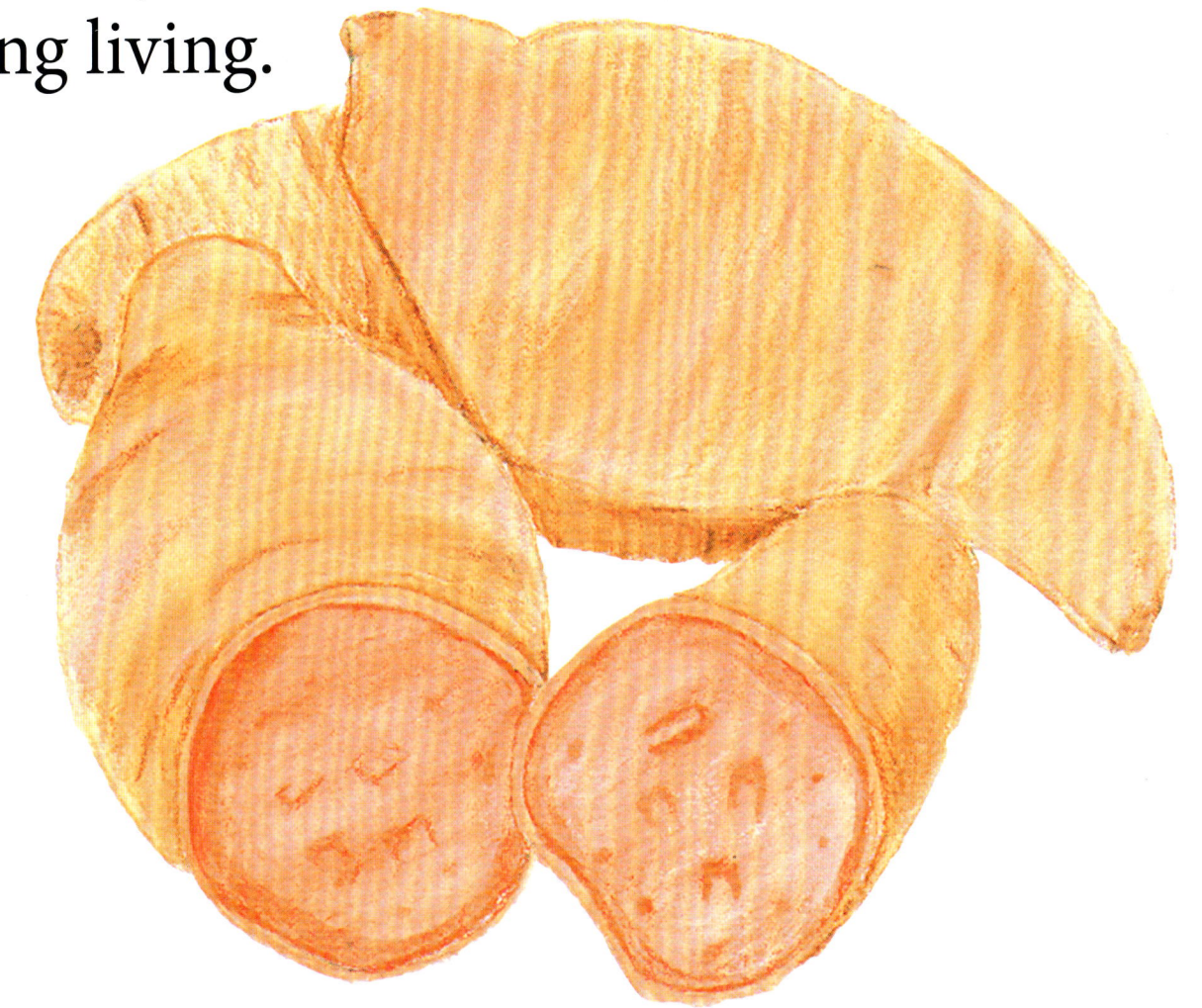

Y is for yams. The smell of yams baking in the oven will remind you of Thanksgiving. You can find them any time of the year, because this root vegetable is long living.

Z

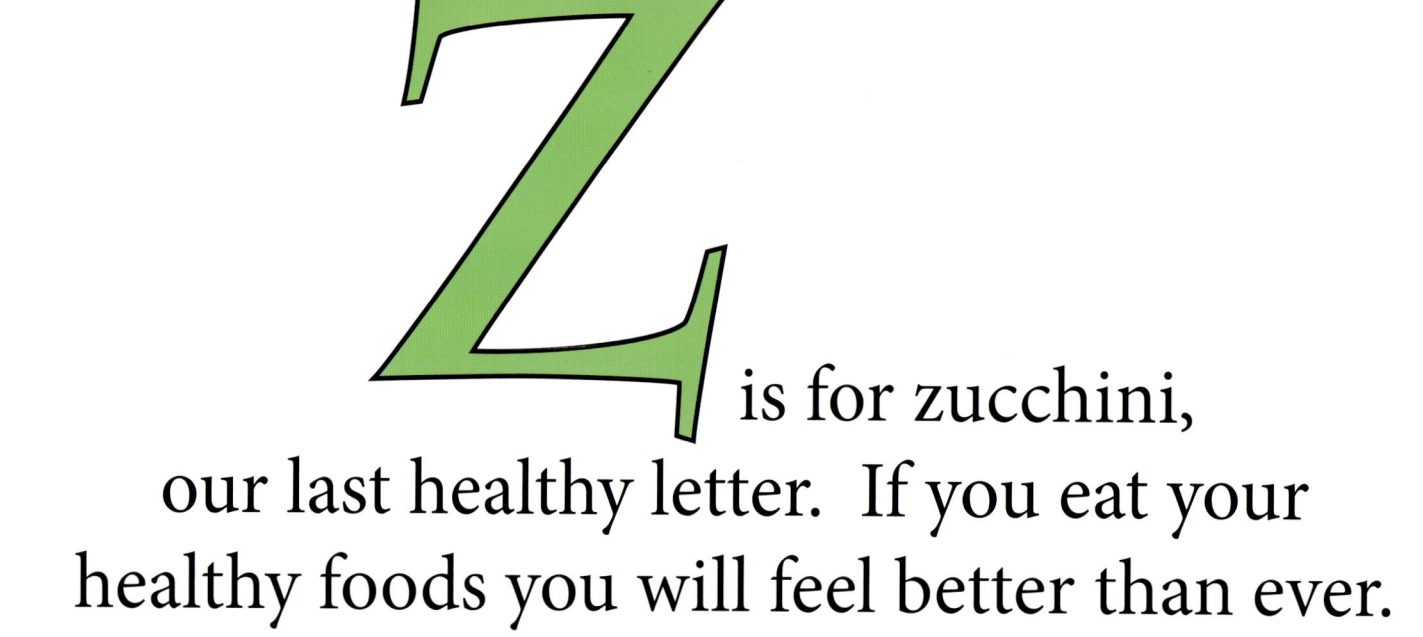

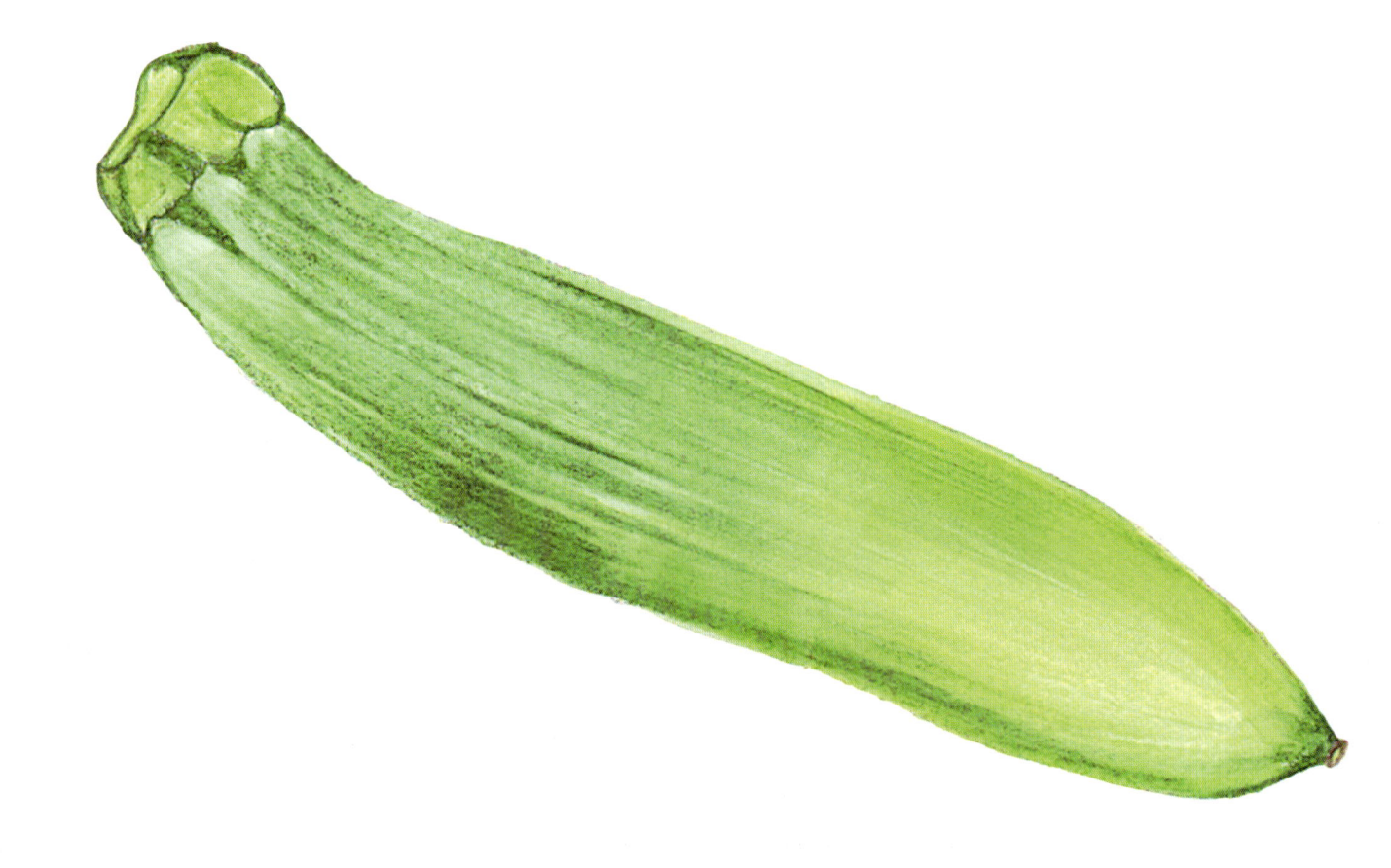

Z is for zucchini, our last healthy letter. If you eat your healthy foods you will feel better than ever.

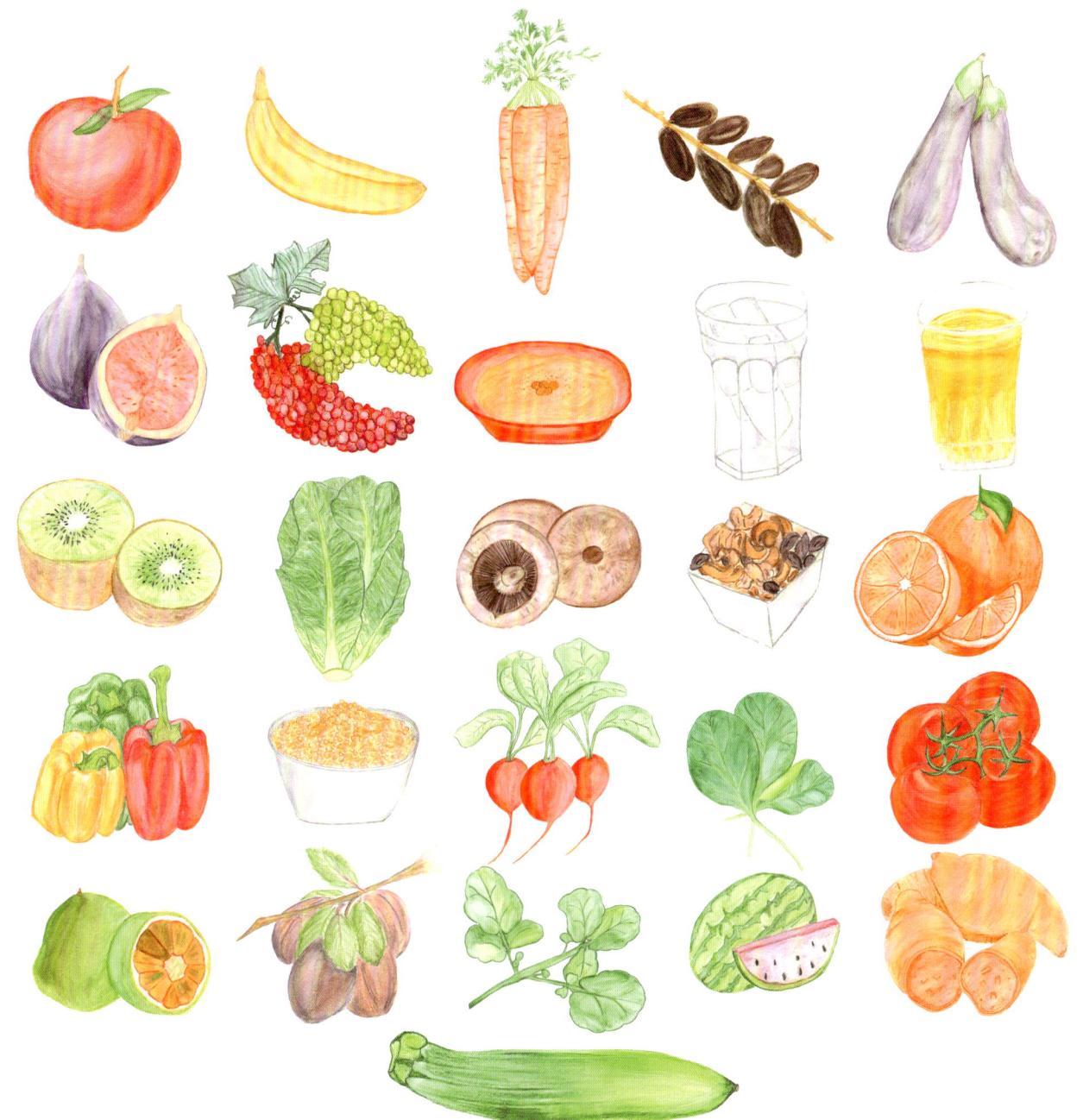

Munch, munch, munch from apple to zucchini. Crunch, crunch, crunch on something healthy at lunch. Now you know your healthy ABCs, so won't you please munch with me?

GLOSSARY

Carbohydrate – This is a main source of energy for your body. Your body changes carbohydrates into blood sugar to give energy to your cells, organs, and tissues. Carbohydrates are found in fruits, vegetables, milk and milk products, whole grain breads, cereal, and legumes (beans and peas).

Fiber – There are two types of fiber. Soluble fiber is partially absorbed in your body and has been shown to lower cholesterol. Insoluble fiber does not dissolve in your body. Insoluble fiber works like a sponge soaking up bad things in your body and brings them out in your waste.

Healthy Fats – Unsaturated fats include polyunsaturated fats and monounsaturated fats. Polyunsaturated fats can be found in nuts, seeds, and fish. Monounsaturated fats can be found in nuts, milk, olive oil, and avocados. These fats have been shown to be good for heart health and for the development of babies inside mommies' tummies.

Herb – An herb is any plant used for flavoring, medicine, or perfume. The herb is the leafy part of the plant, where a spice is usually a dried part of the seed or bark. Some herbs contain great health benefits, such as watercress!

Iron – Iron combines with a protein hemoglobin which helps transport oxygen from your lungs throughout your body. It is an essential mineral. If you don't have enough iron you may feel very tired and weak. Iron also keeps your hair, nails, and skin healthy. This can be found naturally in dried fruit, spinach, beans, and cereal. Iron from meat, poultry, and fish is absorbed two to three times more efficiently than iron from plants.

Magnesium – This mineral is needed to keep good nerve and muscle function, to support a healthy immune system, to keep a good heart beat, and for bone health. It can be found in whole grains, nuts, and dark green leafy vegetables.

Minerals – These are inorganic elements that come from the earth and are absorbed by plants. They are important for your body to stay healthy. A good diet should provide all the minerals you need.

Nutrients - Vitamins and minerals are nutrients that make your body grow and stay healthy.

Phosphorous – A mineral that helps with how the body uses carbohydrates and fats. It also helps the body make protein and store energy. Phosphorous is found in food that is high in protein such as meat, milk, and beans.

Protein – Protein is all over our bodies. It is in every cell, tissue, and organ. It is constantly being broken down and in need of repair. Sources of protein are meat, fish, milk and milk products, eggs, nuts and seeds, tofu, and legumes (beans and peas). The protein we eat is digested into amino acids and then repairs our bodies with the protein we need.

Pulp – This is the texture in your juice when it is not completely strained. It contains fiber.

Sauté – This is a term for a way to cook food in a pan on the stove. Use olive oil for some of those healthy fats!

Superfood – This is a term used to describe food with many health benefits.

Vitamins – These are organic substances that are made by animals or plants. A good diet should provide all the vitamins you need.

Vitamin A – This vitamin helps form healthy skin, teeth, and skeletal and soft tissue. It also produces pigments in the retina of the eye for good eye health. Vitamin A can be found in animal sources such as eggs, meat, fortified milk, and cheese. It is also in bright yellow and orange fruits and vegetables. Another source is leafy greens.

Vitamin C – This vitamin is needed for growth and repair of tissue in your body. All fruits and vegetables contain some amount of vitamin C.

Vitamin K - This vitamin is needed for your blood. Without vitamin K your blood would not clot (which means if you were cut, you would have a hard time to stop bleeding). Some good sources are in green leafy vegetables, meat, eggs, fish, and fortified cereals.